The

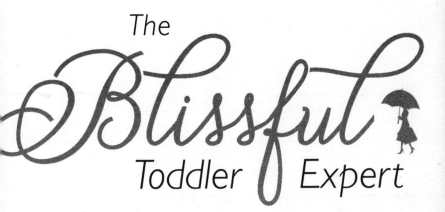

Blissful Toddler Expert

The complete guide to calm
parenting and happy toddlers

LISA CLEGG

Vermilion
LONDON

1 3 5 7 9 10 8 6 4 2

Vermilion, an imprint of Ebury Publishing,
20 Vauxhall Bridge Road,
London SW1V 2SA

Vermilion is part of the Penguin Random House group of companies whose
addresses can be found at global.penguinrandomhouse.com

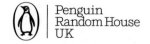

Penguin
Random House
UK

First published by Vermilion in 2015

www.eburypublishing.co.uk

A CIP catalogue record for this book is available from the British Library

ISBN 9780091955007

Printed and bound in Great Britain by Clays Ltd, St Ives PLC

Penguin Random House is committed to a sustainable future for our
business, our readers and our planet. This book is made from
Forest Stewardship Council® certified paper.

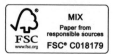

To my husband Martin and our three children Jack,
Ollie and Loren. I love you all to the moon … and back!

Contents

Foreword

When I gave birth to my son in 2011, as a joke my mother gave me her battered and well-worn copy of Dr Benjamin Spock's *Baby and Child Care* book. This had been her bible. She had consulted it on all matters regarding our development as children, and it had given her easy access to guidance. Of course some of the now outdated advice made us laugh, particularly the tip about having a glass of beer or a cigarette to relax you during breastfeeding! With my newborn in my arms, feeling sleep deprived and hormonal, and questioning everything I did as a mother, I knew I needed a modern-day mentor to guide me through those blurry months. I was lucky to come across Lisa early on. She helped in so many ways, I could write a book about it!

My husband and I both have families that live far away, and I didn't have a huge amount of experience of dealing with babies. Lisa gave us confidence as new parents and was a constant source of advice at all hours when we needed it. You have so many questions at the beginning, and the conflicting advice from friends, family, the internet and even strangers is confusing. I think one of the biggest lessons I learnt early on was that there aren't any right or wrong answers, and sometimes it is a matter of trial and error. All children are different, after all. I really valued the fact that Lisa's knowledge and solutions were drawn from her many years' experience as a maternity nurse and a mother of three children. She always said that she planned to write a book, and *The Blissful Baby Expert* has allowed her advice and guidance to be spread far and wide.

Those early months passed quickly, although I am not sure I thought that at the time. Our baby was growing – developing into a little person – and the fact that he was a blissful baby in sleeping, eating and personality was a big help from Lisa.

I hadn't given much thought to the toddler years, but they were quickly upon us. Our little boy was zooming about by 11 months. As always, there were plenty of opinions and advice about what to expect: 'Oh the terrible twos' people would say, or 'Have you potty trained yet?' As a parent, the challenges and development stages change as you start dealing with a talking, walking person who has very strong ideas about what they like, when they like it and how they like it. One of the biggest issues we faced was the battle to get our boy to stay in his 'big boy' bed. He had always slept well in his cot but the freedom to roam around the house at night was too tempting – he was in and out of his new bed like a yo-yo. At my wits' end, I called Lisa and she was again able to guide me with sensible advice on how to tackle this.

One of the most important mantras I learnt from Lisa throughout the baby years, and now toddlerhood, is that as a parent you need 'patience and perseverance' – P&P – for everything. P&P would see me through many a dark night putting my son back to bed, and help me to handle screaming meltdowns as he refused to put clothes on or insisted that he didn't want breakfast. It has meant I don't worry about those issues too much and can really value my time with my son. He makes me laugh at all sorts of things and there is nothing better than a cuddle after a long day at work. He is a blissful toddler, and I am glad that others will get a chance to benefit from Lisa's help through this fascinating stage of a child's life.

Emma Roodhouse, mother to Jacob and Isaac

Introduction

Some of you reading this may have already used the help and advice from my first book *The Blissful Baby Expert*, but now your little one is reaching the toddler years, there will be new challenges ahead. Even if you haven't read my first book, it isn't too late to start implementing changes to work towards a calmer, happier house, using the techniques described in this book.

You will have discovered by now, whether you have read my previous book or not, that I work professionally as a nightly maternity nurse advising parents on all aspects of baby care and development. I have many years' experience working with hundreds of babies and an extremely high success rate advising mums on sleep and feeding issues. Writing *The Blissful Baby Expert* was very easy as I could draw on my experiences with my own three children as babies, as well as my continued professional experience. What, you may ask, gives me the confidence to write a follow-up book based on toddlers?

Well, before I became a maternity nurse I worked as a nanny caring for many toddlers, and I also worked in various day nurseries, again with toddlers. So I have had a lot of professional experience looking after children of that age. On a personal front, I have been through the toddler stage with my three children – and survived! My youngest child, Loren, is going through her toddler years as I write this book, and so I am right in the thick of all the phases that toddlers go through! I'm finding it very helpful as the daily activities and challenges I face with her are ensuring this book covers all of the areas that parents like you will be experiencing too!

When does your little one go from being a baby to a toddler? The term 'toddler' comes from the way that children first walk. Those first uneasy steps are more like a 'toddle' than actual stable, steady walking. There are differing opinions about when this stage begins and ends – it is not solely based on a child's ability to walk. Many would class a toddler as being between the ages of 1–3 years and a pre-schooler between the ages of 3–5 years.

For the purposes of this book, I will be mainly focusing on the 2–4 age group. From time to time I may need to backtrack to the 1–2 age range, to describe or give relevance to certain pieces of information and advice, but I will mostly stick to the experiences and phases you will go through with your child between the ages of 2–4 years.

I'm sure you are wondering how this stage crept up on you so fast. I still can't believe I'm mum to a 12-year-old! Where has your tiny baby gone, whom it feels like you brought home from hospital only yesterday? That cute little baby is now turning into a little person, who has opinions of her own, who pushes you to limits you never thought possible, and who brings you so much joy with her funny words and phrases. This little person once relied on you for everything. As she transitions into a toddler, it will feel like she's pushing you away most of the time as she becomes more independent. She won't want you to do things for her, or even help her at times, and it will positively infuriate her if you try to! If you thought your patience was tried when she was a baby, it will be nothing to the patience you will need as she develops into a little person.

> **TIP**
>
> *The best thing you can give your toddler is time. Toddlers do not like to be rushed. Although I know it is something we as parents sometimes lack, taking the time to be patient can avert a potentially massive toddler meltdown.*

The transition from baby to toddler is a massive step for all of you, with many changes: your toddler will learn to walk, run and climb, feed independently, move from a cot to a bed, toilet train, learn to talk, and start pre-school or nursery. I have divided the book into helpful chapters and sections to guide you along the way.

The toddler years don't have to be stressful. They should be an enjoyable time you spend learning and teaching your toddler new experiences about the world she lives in. Watching her develop every day over these next two years will give you the most amazing sense of pride and achievement that you played the main role in her transition from baby to toddler and beyond.

I hope you all find the information, advice and experiences shared in this book helpful, and that your blissful baby will develop into an equally blissful toddler.

Note: To avoid writing he/she throughout this book, I have alternated the gender of the child in each chapter.

1
Sleep solutions

I believe that the ability to sleep well is a gift for life that you give to your child. Having the right amount of good-quality sleep is essential to wellbeing, whether you're a baby, toddler, child or adult. As a parent, it is part of your job to teach your child good sleeping habits. It is not luck of the draw, as some would suggest, that you either get a 'good sleeper' or a 'bad sleeper'. It is my belief, from all of my experiences both personally and professionally, that you can teach and encourage your child how to settle and sleep well. It is learned behaviour, based on your reactions and the environment you create.

In my experience, a toddler who has always been rocked, cuddled, bottle- or breastfed to sleep, or who has relied on a sleep prop such as a dummy from the baby stage, will not suddenly grow out of needing that comfort without being directed towards settling and sleeping independently.

The problem with relying on sleep props is that each time your toddler passes through his natural sleep cycle and comes into a light sleep, he will realise that the comforter (breast, bottle, dummy, your arms) is no longer there, so he will cry to have it repeated all over again to help him back to sleep. In *The Blissful Baby Expert*, I explain how to teach a baby to self-settle gently, over time, from a young age, by using a good routine and not needing to rely on sleep props. It is not too late to teach good sleeping habits now that your baby is a toddler, if you haven't done it before now.

Sleep cycles

To understand why self-settling is important, you firstly need to understand how sleep cycles work. There are two types of sleep:

Non-Rapid Eye Movement (NREM) or 'quiet sleep'
During the deep state of NREM sleep, blood supply to the muscles is increased, energy is restored, tissue growth and repair occurs, and important hormones are released for growth and development.

Rapid Eye Movement (REM) or 'active sleep'
During REM sleep, the brain is active and dreaming occurs. The body becomes immobile, and breathing and heart rates are irregular. Babies spend 50 per cent of their time in each of these states and the sleep cycle is around 50 minutes. At about six months of age, REM sleep comprises about 30 per cent of sleep. By the toddler years, the sleep cycle is about every 90 minutes. There are four stages of sleep:

1. **Drowsiness:** The eyelids drop and may open and close as your toddler dozes.
2. **Light sleep:** He may move and be startled when he hears a noise.
3. **Deep sleep:** In deep sleep he will breathe deeply and regularly, sometimes with a big sigh. His legs and arms may

move a little or he may suddenly give a start. These sudden movements of the whole body are called 'hypnagogic startles' and are perfectly normal – I'm sure you have experienced them yourself as you drift off into sleep.

4. Very deep sleep: Quiet and not moving.

The usual cycle of sleep starts with stage 1 and then moves through stages 2, 3 and 4. The cycle then moves back through stage 3, then 2 and at this point REM sleep occurs and your toddler may dream. This pattern continues throughout the time your baby is asleep. It is only once they drop into a very deep sleep (stage 4) that they will sleep soundly and won't dream.

The above cycles may occur several times during sleep. A toddler who is unable to self-settle – that is, who cannot settle without the help of a parent or a sleep prop – will be unable to drop into a deep sleep very easily. This means that during the day, toddlers may never sleep for more than one cycle of sleep, sometimes as short as 30–45 minutes. At night it can be slightly longer, but still tends to be a maximum of 90 minutes, although occasionally when toddlers are really exhausted after a few days' unsettled sleep, you may find they sleep for an extended period of time.

If the last thing your toddler remembers as he drifted off to sleep was having a breast, bottle or dummy in his mouth, or being cuddled or rocked to sleep in your arms, then as he drifts back into a light sleep he will understandably be unsettled to realise that comfort has gone. The fact that he is reliant on help to get off to sleep means he will cry for that same comfort each time he passes through the sleep cycle, so roughly every 90 minutes.

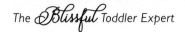

Sleep deprivation

Over time, lack of sleep for both parent and toddler will affect daily life. If a toddler is being given milk to help him settle during the night, whether that is from the bottle or breast, his appetite for food during the day will most definitely be affected (see below).

Interrupted and unsettled sleep will also affect a toddler's behaviour on a daily basis. Sleep deprivation is renowned for making us all short-tempered and impatient with things we may otherwise persevere at.

In my experience, lack of sleep makes toddlers much more clingy and unwilling to be far away from their main carer for any time at all. This lack of independent play can make a transition to nursery or pre-school much more difficult, upsetting and stressful for all of you.

If both you and your toddler are sleep deprived, it won't make for a very happy household. Most parents eventually reach breaking point and decide to ask for help and guidance on how to get their toddler to settle at bedtime and stay asleep all night.

The solutions for your toddler's unsettled sleep will depend on whether he is still in a cot or already in a bed and what the prop is that he is reliant on.

Is your toddler hungry?

A toddler shouldn't be waking from hunger during the night. First and foremost, you need to ensure that your toddler is eating enough during the day, and at the right times (see Chapter 2, pages 42–3), although if the prop he is reliant on to settle at night is the breast or bottle, then his daytime appetite for food will be affected. The aim is to shift his appetite back to the daytime to ensure he gets all of his nutritional needs then, so that he doesn't need to feed at night. You can gradually reduce any night feeds by offering less milk each night. If you are breastfeeding, reduce the time your child is on the breast. If he is reliant on a bottle overnight, either reduce how much milk you put in the bottle, or water it down so it tastes much less appetising, eventually progressing to just a drink of water overnight, if your child wakes thirsty. A toddler should eat three meals per day: breakfast around 7–8am, lunch around 12pm and tea around 5–5.30pm, plus healthy snacks in between if he is eating the meals well. A younger toddler, aged around two, may still be having milk to drink in the morning with breakfast and milk before bed. By around two years old at the latest, you need to transition your toddler to drinking milk from a sippy cup rather than a bottle (see page 53). Firstly, get the morning milk established in a sippy cup, and once your toddler happily drinks at that time from his cup, you can move his bedtime milk to a cup too. This may mean he drinks less milk than he would from the bottle but as long as you offer dairy in other forms to ensure a balanced diet (see page 48), there will be no need to worry. An extra healthy snack, such as a banana before bed, can be offered if you are worried he may wake hungry.

Timed comforting

If your toddler still sleeps in a cot and is reliant on a dummy, milk feed or your presence to help him fall asleep, then I recommend you use timed comforting to encourage him to self-settle (if he sleeps in a bed, see The 'repeat and retreat method', below). The timed comforting technique is about responding to your toddler's needs and offering reassurance,

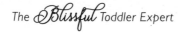

while also encouraging him to self-settle – that is go to sleep without relying on cuddles from you, or a prop such as milk or a dummy. This will ensure he has a better night's sleep. It teaches him that when he wakes up and has a genuine need, you will always come to him straight away. Once you are happy he's not wet, thirsty or in pain, and you have had a nice cuddle for reassurance, then you can encourage him to resettle back to sleep, while continuing to reassure him at the timed intervals.

Depending on the level of speech and understanding your toddler has at two years old, you may be able to briefly explain the plan to no longer allow him to continue having a dummy or bottle to sleep with and that he has to start to settle on his own, without Mummy's help. Keep it simple by saying you think he's a big boy now and his dummies/bottle have to go to the little babies (see also the 'Dummy fairy' section, page 14). If he usually has bedtime milk in the cot or in his room, start giving this downstairs to break the cycle, and then take him to his bedroom for stories and cuddles before bed as a wind-down routine.

The timed comforting method

The timed comforting method incorporates a pat and 'shhh' technique at timed intervals, to reassure your child with your presence, but without actually getting him off to sleep. It encourages him to learn to settle himself.

- Wind your toddler down before bedtime by giving him a bath, a bedtime drink and possibly a snack, reading him a calm story and giving him a cuddle.
- Put him into the cot and give any comforter he likes, such as a muslin or cuddly toy. These are both good sleep props

as, unlike a dummy, they are usually easily found in the night without a parent's help. They tend not to cause unsettled sleep.

- Wind his mobile up if he has one and is used to that, or switch his white noise on, or any music that he has been used to since a baby. *My youngest child is now aged three and we have used a wind-up mobile as her sleep cue from birth. Although the colourful hanging animals are long gone, we now have the wind-up part hanging on a string in her room and still wind it up each night, just before we leave her room at bedtime. If for some reason we are distracted and forget, she will always remind us to do it.*
- Leave the room after giving your toddler a kiss and a cuddle.

If your toddler has been reliant on you cuddling or feeding him until he goes to sleep, or he has a dummy, then this is the point at which he may begin to cry. Wait for two minutes before rushing immediately back in; for some toddlers it is only the initial separation that causes upset and they will stop moaning or crying very quickly and go off to sleep. Many parents find it helpful to use a stopwatch – it ensures they can time the intervals and gives them something to focus on.

If your toddler is upset, return after two minutes and then add two minutes each time to the last time. So the first time he cries go back after two minutes, the second time wait four minutes, the third time six minutes, and so on up to 10 minutes (see below).

- Go back in after two minutes if your toddler is still crying. If he is standing up in the cot, then lie him back down. Pat his back or rub his tummy (depending on if he's sleeping on his front or back) for 15–30 seconds and say 'shhh, sleepy-time', or something similar he understands, and then leave the room again.

- If he cries, wait for four minutes before going back in again. Repeat the pat and 'shhh' as above and then leave again.
- Now if he cries, wait for six minutes and repeat.
- If he cries again, wait for eight minutes and repeat and then 10 minutes and repeat.
- Once you reach the 10-minute interval, you don't need to continue to increase the timings. Stick to 10-minute maximum intervals thereafter unless you feel there is a reason to go in sooner, i.e. your toddler is sick or particularly distressed.

Some parents find it preferable to use longer intervals as going in too often can make some toddlers more distressed, so you have the option of doing five minutes then five minutes, then going straight to 10-minute intervals. It is totally up to you to decide what works best for you and your child. The shorter intervals tend to work best with young babies between 6–12 months but once a child is over 12 months longer intervals may be more effective. It is normal for some toddlers not to calm down when you go in at the timed intervals – some will be infuriated when they don't get what they want. This is the reason some parents prefer to leave the longer intervals as described above.

What you are listening for are gaps and pauses between any crying, instead of persistent, continuous crying. This usually indicates that your toddler will calm and settle down. If the crying isn't continuous, stop going in at the timed intervals at all and allow him to gradually settle himself.

If your toddler's level of crying suddenly increases, then of course you need to go in again, repeat the pat and 'shhh' technique and then leave and resume your timings at the previous interval you got up to – don't start from two minutes again.

The first session of timed comforting is always the hardest and should only be done at bedtime on the first occasion, rather than during a daytime nap. Once your toddler has self-settled once, without his usual sleep prop, such as a dummy, or being fed, cuddled or rocked to sleep, then he will sleep much better than he ever has before. This is because he has settled in the place where he will also come into his light sleep. When he wakes he'll be reassured that he's still in a familiar place that he remembers – his cot – rather than looking for the comforting thing that had helped him fall asleep, such as a cuddle, dummy, bottle or you.

> ### TIP
> *Trust your instinct as to when you go in to reassure your toddler and when it is best to leave him to settle. In the beginning you may have to go in frequently to calm him down. Ultimately, what you are aiming for is that he is calm and self-settles without relying on your presence completely. That will help him to sleep better overnight.*

If your toddler wakes crying a few hours later, go to him straight away to respond and reassure him. You can pick him up, give him a cuddle, check his nappy (or ask if he needs a wee if he's toilet trained) and offer him a drink of water from his cup. If you think teething pain is likely (see page 39), offer pain relief. Once you are reassured he is okay and calm, place him back into his cot and encourage resettling using the timed comforting method again, in the same way you used it before. You may prefer not to pick your child up, and instead offer reassurance while he is in the cot, just trying to pat and 'shhh' him to sleep. Trust your instinct and use the method that helps your child settle most effectively.

Dummy fairy

To help your toddler give up his dummy, I would recommend you use the dummy fairy. There are also various books that you can buy about helping a toddler to stop using a dummy.

Explain to your toddler that the dummy fairy takes away all the dummies from the big girls and boys and passes them on to the small babies who need them. In exchange the dummy fairy leaves a really special present that the child will like. To build up to this, talk to your toddler about the special present he would like to receive as a thank you for giving his dummies to the dummy fairy and the new babies.

On the day you plan to give the dummies away, help your toddler collect them all up and place them in an envelope. Write an address for the dummy fairy on the envelope – a grandparent's or a friend's house will do. The bonus of this age is that they can't actually read what you write!

Walk to the postbox with your toddler and let him post the envelope off to the dummy fairy. If possible, arrange for the special present he has asked for to be there when you return home. When you get home and he discovers the present, make a big fuss about being proud of him and tell him how happy the dummy fairy must have been to see him post off the dummies.

Tell him that the fairy has given him a present as a reward for being such a big, grown-up boy.

Have fun with the present for the rest of the day, as the hard work will start that night when it is time to wind down for bed. That will be when your toddler begins to get tired and may begin to ask for the dummy. At this point you need to stay very calm. If your toddler asks for a dummy, just repeat and remind him that the dummies have gone to the dummy fairy for the little babies and you can't get them back now.

You as parents, maybe even more so than your toddler, need to be ready for the perseverance and consistency that will be needed over the next few days. Don't keep any spare dummies in the house, as you are more likely to relent and give one to your toddler, which will undo all of the preparation stages leading up to this point. If you are consistent, stay calm and repeat yourself, then within 2–3 days he will stop asking for the dummy completely. For the first 24 hours at least, until you get to that stage, you are likely to have a few tears and tantrums and, if your toddler is very clever, he may even suggest you go to the shop to buy him some more dummies!

I used the dummy fairy scenario with my second child, who was the only one out of my three children who had a dummy over the age of 12 weeks. The first night was a tough settling period for an hour or two. I just kept going into his room and reassuring him and once he finally fell asleep for the first time in three years without his dummy, he then stayed asleep all night until 7am. Our first few car journeys were horrendous, as he always used to have a dummy in the car. We had a few days of noisy car journeys where he would be crying and telling me to drive to the shop and buy him some more dummies. He even told me to take his present away and give it back to the dummy fairy so she would bring his dummies back! I refused and stayed calm and said there were no more dummies and I wasn't going to buy him any more. By the end of the week, we had no more tearful car journeys and he was settling and sleeping well at night.

You need to combine the dummy fairy with the repeat and retreat method (see page 18) to encourage your toddler to actually stay in his bed.

Happy wake-up

It is important to encourage self-settling with a happy wake-up routine. This goes a long way to teaching your toddler that he doesn't need to cry in the morning to get you to come. Go to him when he first wakes up happy and chatting (or at least not crying) – don't wait for him to start getting cross and crying. Although it is tempting to have a few extra minutes in bed, it teaches him that crying is the only way to get you to come, so eventually he won't bother waking happy and chatting. Instead he'll go straight to being cross and crying, as he knows that's what gets your attention.

I encouraged this in my children from when they were babies. I have always gone to get them up in the mornings as they were chatting and rolling around the cot happily. I would go in and switch the light on, or open the curtains and greet them with a big 'good morning' smile, which they happily returned. I think it's much nicer to wake up to a happy baby or toddler rather than be greeted bleary-eyed by a screaming toddler every morning. That means you all start off the day in a bad mood.

A happy wake-up will, in turn, mean your child learns to settle to sleep happily. His cot will be seen as a positive place for him to sleep and not somewhere to be feared where he gets ignored.

> **TIP**
>
> *Try using the timed comforting method to settle your toddler for his daytime nap. Most toddlers will still need a 1–2-hour nap minimum, up to the age of at least three years old. Ideally, this should be around midday after lunch. Then ensure he is awake by 3pm so that he settles well at bedtime. If you are consistent with this method, and combine it with the happy wake-up routine, then he will be settling and sleeping much better within a few nights.*

Transitioning from cot to bed

This is a change that many parents naturally worry about, both how and at what age to do it. There is no specific age that you *should* make the transition from cot to bed – only do it once you feel that your toddler is ready. If he is happily settling and sleeping in his cot each night with no regular night-waking and he doesn't make any attempts to climb out, I would advise you leave him to sleep in his cot until he is at least two years old and beginning to develop good language and understanding.

Between the ages of 2–3 years is when you will find the transition to a bed least stressful for all of you, as your toddler will be old enough for you to explain what is happening and to respond to positive praise and rewards for staying in bed. If your toddler is trying to climb out of the cot repeatedly, the transition will need to be done sooner rather than later for safety reasons. A few tips to help the transition:

- Let him choose special bedding that he wants for his new big-boy bed – maybe a favourite book or TV character.

- Explain to him that he's a big boy now and gets to sleep in a bed like some of his friends – make a comparison to one or two of his friends who are already in beds, to make him feel positive about the idea.
- Encourage him to talk about the move to a big bed to family and friends and show visitors his new bed, so they can give praise and positive reinforcement too.
- Think about the timing – don't do the move when your toddler is ill or likely to be a little insecure about other things that are happening – a new baby, starting nursery or toilet training for example.
- Stick to your usual bedtime routine as closely as possible as this consistency will reassure him that the only thing that is changing is his actual bed and he will be more likely to settle down and go off to sleep as he usually does. If he needs extra reassurance then give it but don't be tempted to lie down with him or stay with him until he falls right to sleep, or this will cause settling issues going forward.

The repeat and retreat method, as described below, will be the most effective technique to use, to encourage your toddler to settle well in his new bed and make the transition as smooth as possible.

Repeat and retreat method

If your toddler sleeps in a bed or is about to make the transition from sleeping in a cot to sleeping in a bed, I recommend using the repeat and retreat method. This uses a sticker and reward chart and a wake-up lamp to teach your child to settle at bedtime and want to stay in his bed in the morning until an acceptable time. This approach rewards his efforts and keeps everything calm and positive.

Toddlers have a very determined and persistent energy about them. When they learn that it is very easy to get out of bed, bedtime becomes much easier to resist. If they learn that getting out of bed repeatedly eventually leads to you lying down with them to ensure they stay in bed, or even better, they get to come and snuggle in Mummy and Daddy's bed, then they will be even more determined than ever to wear you down to that point every night.

I know, for some parents, this nightly bedtime battle can be frustrating and tiresome, and at some point, after a particularly challenging evening, you may have got very cross and shouted at your toddler to go to sleep. Shouting and getting cross is never going to make your toddler feel in the mood to go to sleep. In fact, it's more likely to upset him and make the whole settling-down process take much longer. I know I wouldn't be able to relax and go to sleep if someone was getting cross with me and telling me I *had* to go to sleep.

Getting started

To begin the repeat and retreat method:

- **Make a reward/sticker chart:** Buy some interesting stickers, preferably ones related to your toddler's favourite TV characters, or maybe animals he particularly likes.
- **Buy a character lamp:** A small lamp with a 15-watt bulb usually works best. You need to buy a plug-in lamp timer from your local hardware or DIY store – the type that you can plug a lamp into. It will switch the lamp light on automatically at a set time.

Sun/moon clocks

I have found that using a lamp timer works much better than a clock that has a sun/moon face on it, or a picture depicting wake-up time. In my experience, the toddlers whose parents use those have found that their child wakes frequently to check the clock face to see if the sun has come up. Children actually need to wake up and be quite alert to see if the face is a sun or a moon, and they then have to try to get back to sleep again. By the time they come into a light sleep around 5am, it can be very difficult for them to resettle back to sleep so they end up just lying there awake waiting for the clock to change and the novelty wears off pretty quickly.

With the lamp timer, your toddler doesn't actually need to be awake fully to know if the lamp is on or not – it will be pretty obvious, even when he is drowsy, if a light is on in his room. Many parents who have come to me for advice have been using something similar to a sun/moon clock successfully, but eventually found that the novelty of the clock has worn off and their toddler is waking earlier and earlier each morning. When I advise they change to the lamp timer solution, it works very quickly and combined with the reward chart and retreat and repeat method, their toddler is soon sleeping better again.

Once you have all of the build-up stages in place and have explained the concept to your toddler, the next stage is implementing it all:

- **On the day that you plan to start the new routine,** have everything ready and in place – the reward chart and the lamp set up in your toddler's room.

- **Set the lamp for an achievable and acceptable time:** If your toddler has regularly been waking and getting up at 4 or 5am, then set the lamp timer to 6am to start with. It can be gradually pushed closer to 7/7.30am by changing the timer and setting the lamp to come on 10–15 minutes later every three days, as long as your toddler is happily achieving the current wake-up time you have set.
- **Make sure you have a calm period leading up to bedtime:** Give him a bath, let him watch a little bit of relaxing children's TV and then go up to his bedroom for a story or two.

TIP

Negotiate how many stories you will read – one or two – and don't let your toddler use the idea of requesting more stories to keep you in the room longer and delay you leaving.

- **Explain to him that you want him to stay in his bed** and go to sleep and in the morning he needs to wait for the lamp to come on. Tell him that when the lamp comes on it is time to wake up and have breakfast. Once the lamp is on then he can call you to come and get him up, or come into your room to wake you up. Tell him that if he needs to go to the toilet (if he's toilet trained), he can call you but if he gets out of bed in the night for anything else you will take him back to bed each time. Remind him that he's a big boy now and use any siblings, or older cousins or friends, as examples of people who stay in their own beds all night until morning. He has to stay in his own bed all night and not have you lying next to him until he falls asleep, to be able to earn the sticker in the morning.

- **Each time he gets out of bed,** after you have tucked him in for the final time, you should pick him up, carry him back to bed calmly and as you put him in bed say something like, 'It's bedtime, Mummy loves you.' Don't get cross, don't deviate from the simple words you choose – keep things simple and boring and repeat the message each time he gets out of bed.

- **Be consistent and persevere:** sticking to the same words and putting your toddler back to bed will be what makes this method work. If, when he gets out of bed, you have a whole conversation with him about staying in bed and why, you are giving him lots of attention for his behaviour and that will make him want to continue to get out. However, if you make the idea of getting out of bed very boring – don't enter into conversation, just continue putting him back every time, then eventually he will think, 'What's the point in getting out? They only put me back again each time!'

- **In the morning let him choose a sticker to go on his reward chart** for being so clever and waiting for the light. Have a system that if he gets three stickers, you will plan a trip to the park or something similar that he likes doing. For five stickers in a row, then he gets a bigger treat.

The idea is to encourage your toddler to *want* to stay in bed by positively reinforcing his good behaviour. Anything else should be ignored. No matter how many times he gets out of bed in the evening and night and you have to put him back, you must reward the fact that eventually he resettled without you staying with him and did, in fact, wait for the light – give huge praise for doing that. If he's used to coming into your bed, having a dummy or is used to you lying or sitting with him to help him to go to sleep, any night where that doesn't happen is already an improvement and should therefore be rewarded, even if you had to go in several times to put him back to bed and reinforce the message.

If your toddler knows he gets rewarded for waiting for the light, after a few nights when he comes into a light sleep he will stir, see that the light isn't on and resettle himself without needing to call you until it's morning and the light comes on. He will learn that he makes you very happy by doing that.

> **TIP**
>
> *It's very important that both parents are consistent with this method and use exactly the same words and process. If you would like to take it in turns, then of course that's fine, but rather than putting him back only one time each, I would suggest you set timed intervals you work towards. For example, Mummy does the repeat and retreat method for a 10–20 minute period constantly and then Daddy does it. This should be the same in the night. It will be too unsettling if you literally take it one turn each.*

The first night will of course be the hardest for all of you. Just repeat the process of putting your toddler back each time at bedtime until he settles. In the night when he wakes for the first time, you should check he's okay initially and doesn't need anything – for example, a drink, the toilet, that he's not too hot or cold, or scared from a bad dream. Once you have established and satisfied any need, praise him for sleeping so

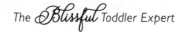

well up to now, reassure him and then remind him to wait for the light to come on in the morning to call you to wake up too.

Leave the room once you have tucked him in and it is at this point that you should begin the repeat and retreat method if he continues to get out of bed. Put him back each time he gets out and say something like, 'Sleepy-time – wait for the light.' If he doesn't actually get out, but instead stays in his bed crying, you can use the timed comforting technique (see page 9) to keep going back to lie him down and reassure and repeat, 'Sleepy-time – wait for the light.'

In the morning when he wakes and calls you to tell you that the light has come on, you should heap lots of praise on him, no matter how many times he woke previous to that and you had to put him back in bed. Make a big fuss about him calling you when the light came on and tell him how clever he is. Let him choose one of his new stickers for the chart and remind him again that when he has three, then you will take him on a special trip to the park (or a similar activity that he enjoys). When he gets five stickers, you can offer a bigger treat.

If you give lots of positive praise, then he will respond to that very quickly. This method has been used by so many of the parents who email me every day and if the directions are followed and implemented correctly then you will begin to see improvements within three days.

CASE STUDY: Natasha and Jack

Jack was three-and-a-half when his mother Natasha contacted me. Jack had never been a good sleeper and when Natasha was three months pregnant with her second child and still sleeping on Jack's bedroom floor, she decided it was time to seek help. Natasha and her husband Phil had always found it difficult to settle Jack. He always seemed to find ways to keep them in his bedroom at bedtime, despite the strict bedtime routine they had established – bath, story and bed.

Jack woke frequently in the night and called out crying or went into his parents' room. A health visitor initially suggested sitting with Jack until he settled, moving further away from him every 2–3 days. This was advised to ensure he was feeling totally secure when he fell asleep. This method is known as 'gradual retreat' by many health professionals and sleep experts and, despite it having been successful for some parents and children, this technique actually made Jack regress even more. He became insecure about when Mummy or Daddy would leave him, and would desperately try not to go to sleep at all, for fear of them eventually leaving the room. Once he finally did fall asleep, he would wake again 30–60 minutes later when he came into a light sleep and call for Mummy or Daddy and they would have to go and lie with him again to resettle him.

This has always been my experience of parents who have been advised to try this method. It tends to work initially but as soon as the parents get to the point they are sitting by the door or outside the door, the toddler becomes very insecure again that they can't actually see Mummy or Daddy. The parent then has to move closer to the bed again to help the child resettle.

At the point Natasha called me she was curled up outside Jack's room several times per night with a pillow and duvet, to resettle him and he would call out to her every now and then to check that she was still there. If at any point she didn't answer him because she had crawled back to her own bed, he would get up and come and wake her again to repeat the whole process all over again. Being pregnant with her second child, Natasha was even more exhausted and knew that she couldn't let things continue the way they were and that was when she contacted me.

I explained the repeat and retreat method to Natasha. I warned her that it would be very difficult for the first couple of nights, in particular, and Jack would test her and her husband Phil to the limit. However, as long as they stuck to repeatedly putting him back to bed each time and didn't resort to sleeping with him or letting him into their bed again, he would very quickly get the idea of the new bedtime routine.

This quote below is from Natasha herself:

'Given the history, Lisa advised the repeat and retreat method, which was to immediately direct Jack back into bed without entering into any conversation. This was initially very hard to do as Jack was crying and desperately seeking some kind of communication with Mummy or Daddy, regardless of what time of the night it was. We would always give a cuddle and reassure him when he first woke up and make sure he was okay, and then we tucked him back into bed and began putting him back each time he got out. We initially said, "Night night, love you," the first couple of times we returned him to bed but in the end we found it was better not to say anything at all to him. One night he was returned to his bed over 300 times (this is not an exaggeration, I promise). That night was the worst – he was angry and frustrated with us and cried, which broke our hearts, but we knew we had to persevere for all of our sakes as we couldn't physically cope with the disrupted nights any more, and knew it wasn't good for Jack.

The second night was much better and the third one better again, and we finally felt we had taken control of the situation. After a couple of weeks we started having a full night's sleep for the first time since Jack had been born. Even now Jack has a tendency to sometimes wake and after reassuring him and making sure he's okay, we stick to the same routine and we never let things get out of control like before.'

The repeat and retreat method is very effective and will encourage your toddler towards better sleeping habits, but it takes hard work to get there. If your toddler has been reliant on your presence completely for every bedtime and naptime and has repeatedly woken in the night for more than two years, it will not be easy to turn things around. However, be reassured that it is not impossible. As long as your child feels comforted and you respond to him, then he will eventually settle down. The wake-up lamp and the reward chart are an important part of encouraging your toddler to settle without you sitting with him all the time. It should be a positive experience so he feels reassured and *wants* to stay in his bed in order to earn your praise and reward in the morning. If you focus on that, then you will all soon be enjoying undisturbed sleep again.

Should you use a stair gate?

For most parents who end up using a stair gate on their child's bedroom door, the decision is usually based on the safety of their child. Bedtime is about teaching your child how to happily settle to sleep without relying on your presence. Putting a stair gate on the bedroom door can be a good idea once your toddler makes the transition from cot to a bed, if he is the type of child who may wander around the house at night, rather than come to your room to wake you.

The stair gate can be a good bargaining tool for you: agree with your child that you will take the stair gate off when he can agree to stay in his bed all night and wait for the lamp to come on, without always coming out.

We didn't use a stair gate initially when any of our three children moved from a cot to a bed. We have two cats so have always shut our children's bedroom doors to prevent the cats going into their rooms at night. However, my husband is a very heavy sleeper and doesn't always hear our children wake

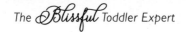

in the night, when I am out of the house at work in my job as a maternity nurse. Our eldest was under two years old when he moved to a bed as he began literally launching himself out of his cot every night repeatedly, while still in his Grobag – don't even ask me how he managed that!

The house we lived in had very steep stairs and he still insisted on wearing his Grobag in his big-boy bed, so we decided a stair gate on his bedroom door was the safest option to prevent him possibly falling down the stairs in the night if he woke and came looking for us.

Our second son has inherited a lovely family trait from his uncles of sleepwalking! He wanders around the house half asleep and remembers nothing of it in the morning, so we put the stair gate on his bedroom door to keep him safe. At eight years old now, he still wakes 2–3 times per night to go to the toilet and occasionally we discover strange things he has done overnight that he has no clue about. My husband prevented him going to the toilet in the corner of his older brother's room by mistake one evening, thankfully. His most recent sleepwalking episode meant he woke in the morning naked and wasn't quite sure why, until he went to go to the toilet and discovered his pyjama bottom trousers there! He must have put them in the toilet in the night for some reason and didn't remember a thing.

Our youngest child initially transitioned well from her cot to a bed but then became very ill with a bad cough, cold, tonsillitis and a chest infection, which lasted a couple of weeks. During this time her sleep was understandably disrupted and we had to get up to her frequently to give her extra medicine and offer her regular drinks of water. She also slept in with us quite a lot so we could keep an eye on her as she was so poorly.

Once she was better again, we had to convince her that she must settle and sleep in her own bed all night and Mummy's and Daddy's bed was no longer an option. We found putting the stair gate on her door did the trick in the end as she wouldn't be able to wander around the house without our knowledge. Putting a lamp on a timer also motivated her to sleep all night and proudly call us in the morning when the lamp came on.

A good bedtime routine

A good wind-down routine is essential to relax your toddler for bedtime. Ensure that he has a short nap over the lunchtime period so that he's not overtired at bedtime. Bath him and do some calm activities afterwards – for example, do a puzzle or let him watch some low-key television. A drink of warm milk and a small snack can also ensure you don't have any hunger complaints as soon as it's time to head upstairs. Toilet time and teeth brushing should be first and then take him to his bedroom and read one or two stories. Have a cuddle, remind him to wait for his 'wake- up lamp' to come on in the morning and then say goodnight.

> **TIP**
>
> *Your toddler will be reassured by having a consistent bedtime routine.*

Nightmares and common night-time fears

As a toddler, your child is learning so many new things every single day, and new experiences can sometimes lead to fears that affect bedtime. Your toddler's imagination is amazing

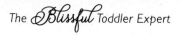
at this age, which is great for playtime, but it may lead him to being scared of all manner of things when he is alone in his room.

The dark

Despite the fact that your toddler has always slept in a dark room, he may now be requesting to have a light on. Buy a small night-light that isn't too bright – only 10–15 watt – a lamp with a picture of a favourite TV or book character on it might go down well. Leave it on to reassure him once you've said goodnight. Alternatively, leaving the landing light on may be enough to reassure him. This light needs to be separate to the wake-up lamp you have on a timer, to let your toddler know that it is an acceptable time to get up (see pages 19–24). To make the idea effective, the wake-up lamp should serve one purpose only; it shouldn't be used for anything else.

Leaving the bedroom door open

Your toddler may start asking for the bedroom door to be open when previously he was happy to have it closed. For us as a family, having the door open isn't an option because we have cats that will go into the bedrooms at night and try to sleep on the children's beds. If my toddler asks to have her door open, I just remind her of this fact and say I will leave her lamp on instead. She's always reassured by that.

If you are happy to leave your toddler's door open slightly to reassure him, it's fine as long as he promises to stay in his bed. You could come to an agreement that you will leave the door open, but if he starts to get out of bed then you will have to close it.

Monsters and scary things under the bed!

This is more likely to be a fear that your toddler has nearer to the age of four years old – it is around this time that his imagination will really begin to run wild. Try to be aware of any TV programmes he may be watching that could be creating or adding to any fear, particularly any he has watched right before bedtime – and limit TV time to very relaxing, calm programmes before bed.

Make sure the bedtime story that you read doesn't have a storyline involving capturing or chasing anyone. Older siblings can also be unhelpful and can create a fear at bedtime by playing chasing games, pretending to be monsters, or even using their favourite Halloween masks to scare their younger sibling. Aim for a very calm, relaxed bedtime routine (see above) to wind your toddler down, so he's more likely to settle easily.

Nightmares

It is fairly common for toddlers and pre-school children to wake up scared after having a nightmare, as their imagination runs wild. In most cases it happens infrequently and reassuring your toddler, when it does happen, will be enough to calm him. Allow him to talk about what happened in his dream if he wants to and reassure him with cuddles, before encouraging him to settle back down in his own bed. Don't be tempted to bring him into your bed – bad habits are easily formed and if he knows that coming into your bed is an option, he may begin to wake more frequently at night to see if he can snuggle in with you. Reassure him, cuddle him, and then resettle him in his own bed. Try to leave the room before he falls back to sleep relying on your presence, so that he is able to self-settle after your reassurance.

If nightmares are a more regular occurrence and begin to happen every or most nights, then it can indicate that your child is stressed about something. It may be something big like the death of a relative or a family breakdown, or linked to a change such as a new baby sibling, starting school or nursery, or moving house. Encourage your toddler to talk to you about anything he is worried about and reassure him as much as you can. To help prevent nightmares:

- Make sure the bedtime routine (see page 29) is calm, relaxed and the same each evening.
- Don't feed your toddler too close to bedtime as that can keep the metabolism working hard, which in turn keeps the brain active. Bedtime is the point of the day when you need to keep things calm and decrease brain activity.
- Don't let him watch scary or action-packed TV programmes or bedtime stories right before you want him to go to sleep. Stick to simple, calm books or programmes.

TIP

It is better to recognise and acknowledge and appropriately deal with any fears your toddler tells you about. If you dismiss them as silly, they are more likely to develop into a much larger fear that affects his sleep badly.

Night terrors
Night terrors typically occur in children from the ages of 3–12 years, with the peak age for them starting being three-and-a-half years old. Between 1–6 per cent of children experience night

Monster spray

If your child regularly worries or talks about monsters or other scary things that he believes are in his room at night, introduce the 'Mummy monster spray'. Fill a simple spray bottle with plain water and add a few flower petals or a touch of glitter to jazz the spray up a bit.

Tell your toddler that your special spray will send all bad things away and make his room a happy place for him to sleep. You could even use the monster spray in your bedroom and any siblings' rooms to reinforce the idea and reassure your toddler – turn it into a very relaxed, fun game. As you spray, say something like, 'Go away scary things, we don't want you,' and then reassure him once you have sprayed each room by telling him that he doesn't need to be scared any more.

terrors at some stage, with both boys and girls and children of every race being affected. They are usually something that your child will just grow out of, although sometimes you can prevent or stop them altogether. As explained on page 6, sleep is divided into two categories: REM (Rapid Eye Movement sleep) and Non-REM sleep. Non-REM sleep is then further divided into four stages.

Night terrors typically occur during the transition from stage three Non-REM sleep to stage four, and usually happen around 90 minutes after your child has initially gone to bed and fallen asleep. A night terror is completely different from a nightmare, which happens during REM sleep. During a night terror your child will be crying intensely and be genuinely scared of something and seem awake, but at the same time be unable to recognise you or be calmed by your presence. You may also notice, as you are trying to calm him, that his heart rate and breathing are increased and he may take much longer before he relaxes and sleeps normally again.

Night terrors are difficult for a parent to witness, as you will feel completely out of control and unable to reassure your child and just have to wait until it ends. Most children do not remember the night terror the next day, unlike a bad dream. Night terrors can be triggered by certain things:

- Stressful life events, such as the death of a relative, or a change to family home life and dynamics.
- Fever (see page 237): If your toddler has a very high temperature, he may become delirious and hallucinate.
- Sleep deprivation: Ensure your toddler has a nap or at least a rest midway through the day and isn't overtired when you put him to bed.
- Recent anaesthesia for surgery.
- Certain medications that affect the brain.

No medical treatment is available to stop night terrors. Instead parents are advised to take the following precautions:

- Maintain a relaxed and consistent bedtime routine and wake-up time.
- Make your child's room safe, so that if he does have a night terror he will not injure himself.

The most common form of trying to prevent and stop night terrors is to interrupt your toddler's sleep over a period of a few days. In 90 per cent of night terror cases, this preventative waking usually stops night terrors occurring any more.

1. Take a note of how many minutes after your child falls asleep that the night terror usually occurs.
2. Wake your child up 15 minutes before the night terror usually occurs and keep him awake and out of bed for five minutes. It's usually a good idea to take him to the toilet to see if he would like to go.
3. Continue waking him as described above for seven nights in a row.
4. On the eighth night, do not wake him and see what happens.

CASE STUDY: Lisa and Charlie

This is a case study from a mum who contacted me about her son Charlie, who was having night terrors. The following statement was written by Charlie's mum, Lisa:

'My son Charlie has always been a deep sleeper. He has always loved his sleep and he has always dreamed during sleep, too. It was not unusual to hear him talking in his sleep – in fact, it was a regular occurrence. In the autumn of one year, when he was almost three years old, he began to have night terrors. They were absolutely awful – 90 minutes after I put him to bed every night, he would wake up screaming, clearly scared to death, telling us he couldn't find his Mummy and Daddy. It was heartbreaking to watch and was taking longer and longer to calm him down each night, so I contacted Lisa for advice just before Christmas.

Lisa advised me to wake Charlie 15 minutes before an episode would usually start. I also had to make sure we took him to the toilet, so he was fully awake and then put him back to bed. We did this for five nights and it stopped any night terrors occurring that week. On the

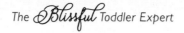

sixth night we decided not to wake him and see what happened – he slept soundly and hasn't had one night terror since! All in all a happy Charlie and happy Mummy and Daddy thanks to Lisa.'

Different routines while away from home

If your toddler attends a childcare setting such as nursery, pre-school or a childminder's, or he goes to a relative's house on certain days each week, then you may find that his routine has to be adapted to suit. Your childcare provider may find it difficult to stick to your toddler's usual schedule. In a nursery setting, in particular, mealtimes have to coincide with all of the other children at a set time each day. Your toddler's naptime is also very likely to be different, if he still has one. For many toddlers, the excitement of being in a different, more social environment with so much going on, means they may not even want to sleep at all, despite the childcare provider's best efforts to convince them to.

Depending on how long and often your toddler goes, this can be an advantage or disadvantage. A parent's biggest task can sometimes be keeping a toddler awake on the journey home at 5 or 6pm, if he is doing a full day. If a toddler falls asleep at that time, it can mean that bedtime ends up being quite late and you have to battle with a grumpy overtired toddler. On those days, you just have to go with the flow and adapt the usual bedtime routine accordingly.

If your toddler attends some kind of childcare setting on only a couple of days per week, you may find that he adapts very well between the different routine times of naps and meals – he may even enjoy a longer sleep at home on 'Mummy days' to catch up from the exhaustion of nursery days (that's what happens with my toddler). If he attends more regularly, it's sometimes easier to adapt your routine so that it is similar to the nursery one, to allow his body to get used to it on a regular basis.

Holidays

So many parents contact me asking how they can maintain their toddler's routine while on holiday, without it restricting them too much and spoiling the enjoyment of the break away. My answer is always the same: while on holiday or away from home, for the most part, you have to go with the flow and find a routine that suits your holiday. Like most people, you may find the evenings when your toddler would usually be tucked up in bed sleeping are nice to spend exploring or going out to dinner or dancing with friends.

An overtired, fractious toddler will not make that an enjoyable experience for anyone so it is important you encourage a late afternoon nap if you want to have a more relaxed evening each night. The first 24 hours are always difficult as your toddler misses out on a few hours' sleep through travel and arriving early or late. By the following day though, he should be tired enough for you to begin to establish a good daytime sleep, so that he has the energy to last into the evening with a later bedtime.

My toddler usually wakes around 7/7.30am, naps from 12.30–3pm and goes to bed around 7.30pm when we are at home. Last year we went to Tenerife and we adapted her routine to suit us. Our routine when we went away was supper in the restaurant around 7pm; party games and dancing in the family club-house until 11pm–12am; back to the apartment where our toddler would settle into the travel cot straight away and then we would wake her at 9/9.30am each day to go and have breakfast.

We would then have lunch around 1pm when the restaurant opened and after lunch I would go back to the apartment with her on our own and we would have a snooze together – it was a bonus that I got to sleep too from 2–5/5.30pm. We would then wake her and give her a bath or shower and go out for dinner again at 7pm.

This was a routine that worked well for us while we were away. It took a few days when we got home for her to adjust back to her usual home routine of naptimes and bedtimes, but with a few days of good old patience and perseverance, she soon settled down.

Despite the fact that your toddler may happily self-settle to sleep at home, don't be surprised if he needs extra attention and reassurance to help him settle when you are in a new environment that he is not used to. This may involve you sitting next to the cot or bed as he falls asleep, lying in the bed next to him for reassurance, or allowing him to fall asleep in the pushchair and then transferring him to the cot or bed.

Many parents worry that by giving this extra help and reassurance while on holiday, their toddler is likely to slip into bad sleep habits and need the same help all the time once they are home. In my experience with my own three children and holidays, and from chatting to lots of other parents, as long as you are consistent on your return and go back to your usual bedtime and nap routine as soon as possible, then your toddler will very quickly settle down again. It may take a few days or even a week, depending on the time difference if you went on holiday abroad and any jet lag your toddler may be experiencing. As with everything with babies and toddlers – patience and perseverance is the key. If you are struggling to get your toddler to settle back into the home routine again, you may need to implement the 'repeat and retreat method' method (see page 18).

Teething and illness

These are the two things that are always going to cause unsettled or disrupted sleep. Your toddler will have his canines and molars cutting any time between the ages of 1–3 years, and these are the most painful teeth to cut. The molars, in particular, have to cut on all four corners, as they are so big, so can cause weeks of grumpiness, food refusal and night waking. If your toddler has good speech developing, then hopefully he may be able to indicate teething pain to you, so that you can offer relief accordingly.

Anbesol teething liquid is the product I have found particularly effective at relieving pain. Infant ibuprofen products are also much more effective on any kind of pain than infant paracetamol products. Always follow the guidance on the packaging.

Whether he is ill or teething, your toddler will need extra cuddles and reassurance during the day and even night. He is likely to be much more clingy to you and even if he usually self-settles to sleep, he may struggle to do that. Go with the flow until you are sure he is well again or over his teething bout, and any bad sleeping habits formed can soon be discouraged and self-settling achieved with the two Ps – patience and perseverance!

All toddlers have the ability to settle and sleep well if they are taught good habits and encouraged to settle happily, with reassurance when needed and by being given consistent boundaries. I have helped hundreds of parents who have emailed me via the free advice service I provide, many of whom are at their wits' end with a toddler who has either never been a good sleeper according to them, or has fallen into bad habits due to illness, a new sibling arriving or because of a transition from a cot to a bed. Using the methods described in this chapter consistently, I've helped many parents teach their toddler how to settle to sleep independently and sleep well with praise and encouragement, and that is a massive gift that all the family can enjoy!

2

Feeding your toddler

As a baby your child may have been a fantastic eater with a good appetite and been willing to eat anything and everything. For some parents this ease will continue into toddlerhood – if you are one of these lucky ones, then congratulations! For the majority of us, however, some effort will have to be put in, and lots of encouragement given, to ensure our children remain eating a varied and balanced diet.

As your little one moves from being a baby to a toddler, she will learn that what and how much she eats is about the only thing in her life she can fully control. If she is tired, you can put her to bed, even if sometimes she protests. You know she is tired, so you persevere. If she throws something or hits someone, you can take the toy away or put her in some sort of time out. When it comes to food and eating, it is totally different. If your toddler doesn't want to eat, you can't force her to. Could anyone force you? Babies and toddlers learn pretty quickly that this choice they have about food could be a major advantage to them, if you let it get to that stage. As long as you are consistent in your rules where good eating habits are concerned, then you won't ever have a child that becomes too fussy with food.

Fussiness with food

Illness and teething are likely to affect your toddler's appetite: she may go off her food and become fussy about the food she eats when she is dealing with these discomforts. They can be the start of the slippery slope into food fussiness and refusal to eat foods that were previously enjoyed. If your toddler has had a sore throat, for example, you may have been giving her softer foods to eat or allowed her to dictate what she wanted to eat, just so you felt reassured that at least she was eating something. If you don't rein this control back your way once she is better, though, it can very quickly progress from initial fussiness to more complex eating problems.

As a parent, one of your biggest worries is likely to be whether your child is eating enough. This begins at the newborn stage when you are breast- or bottle-feeding and getting your baby weighed regularly, and continues to the day your child leaves home! Actually it probably doesn't even stop then – my mum is always trying to give me way too big a portion when we visit, and I'm 34! She's also always checking if I've fed my own three children (I have, in case you were wondering!)

At times, particularly when children are ill and they have a reduced appetite or just don't want to eat anything, it is very difficult to sit back and wait. You just want them to eat! It's a natural parental feeling and reaction. If they eat, they might have more energy and feel better, right? The thing to try to remember, and keep reminding yourself, is that it is highly unlikely that your child will ever starve herself. I know it is not an experiment you will ever want to try as a parent, but you have to give your toddler a little bit of responsibility if she is ill or teething. Children know if they feel like eating, they know how hungry they feel and, if you pressure them too much, then you create a bad association with food and make them even less likely to want to eat, even once they feel well again!

As I write this, my toddler has been ill with a virus for two days – she has a high temperature and horrible hacking cough. Do you know what she has eaten today in total? Half a cookie! I'm being serious! I have offered her various things throughout the day but she has refused everything. She has spent the day sleeping off the germs trying to invade her body and the last thing she needs is me pressuring her to eat! Would I like her to eat? Of course! But I know that she knows how she feels and if she doesn't want to eat today then that's fine, as long as she's drinking some fluids. I know in a few days' time when she feels much better, her appetite will pick up and she will want to eat again. I can then begin to encourage good food choices.

> **TIP**
> Always try to remember, the natural instinct to eat when hungry will always outweigh any stubbornness your child has over food refusal.

Sweet versus savoury foods

Most babies show a preference for sweet foods over savoury offerings from the first weaning tastes you offer them. Sweet is a natural choice for most children and even adults – most of us when offered the choice between some crackers and cheese or a slice of cake, choose the sweet pudding.

I've never minded my children eating sweet things, as long as they understand it is a treat that they can have only *after* they have eaten their main meal. I encourage parents to teach this habit to their children as early as possible, as I did – from those first stages of weaning is the ideal time. The savoury meal should always come before any pudding and if the baby refuses this, no sweet or pudding is offered.

How to implement this with a baby is explained in more detail in my book *The Blissful Baby Expert*. If you have not read that and used the tips when your toddler was a baby, then it is *not* too late to start now she is a toddler.

You need to get to the stage where pudding time or the chance to have a sweet treat is left in your toddler's hands – or at least seems to be! The way to do this is by providing small manageable portions of savoury and fruit courses that you know your child's appetite can cope with. Offering your toddler a portion of food that is far too big might put her off even attempting to eat it. Small portions and good eating habits are much easier to reward.

If you were to put all of the vegetables, carbohydrates and protein sources of their main meal into a big pile, then the initial portion size you offer should be no bigger than an adult's clenched fist. Obviously, some toddlers will happily eat double or even triple this quantity if they have a larger appetite. However, if you base your initial serving on this portion size, it gives your toddler a choice to ask for more once she has finished. If you hand some of the responsibility to your toddler, she will feel less pressured and will be more likely to eat with no fussing or silliness. It will also make *you* less stressed and worried about the amount that she is eating.

Sweet treats and unhealthy snacks

Outside influences from other children and even adults can affect how well your toddler eats on a day-to-day basis. If you go out to lunch and take a picnic, it is a certainty that your toddler will be interested to see what her friends have for their lunch and compare it to her own food. Depending on how well you know the people you lunch with, you can agree that the toddlers can share different parts of their lunch if they would like to, in order to keep everyone happy.

Recently we went to the zoo with friends and my toddler had a small chocolate bar as her treat for after her sandwiches and fruit, and the other toddler we were with had some crisps. Of course, my toddler wanted crisps and the other one wanted the chocolate, because they were drawn to something they didn't have. To keep everyone happy, the other mum and I split the chocolate and the crisps in half, so both toddlers got both and everyone was happy. If you don't have the option of splitting the lunch boxes for the toddlers to share, agree to give your toddler a treat when you get home if she eats what she has in her lunch box while out. Here are some other ways to handle your toddler's love of sweet treats:

- At home, keep sweets and treats out of reach of your toddler. Many are often fully aware of where the treats are kept and will happily help themselves to them if you are distracted for any length of time.
- Most grandparents love to spoil their grandchildren and often do so by offering them sweets and treats. If you are present, you can make it clear that you don't want your toddler to have any sweets until after their lunch or supper, if it is imminent. If you have left your toddler solely in her grandparents' care, it will be very difficult to control what she eats. *I know my children pretty much eat whatever they want when they go to my parents, and that most of it is*

pretty unhealthy. Although my mum knows I don't like it, she chooses not to follow my instructions and instead relents to the pleading of her grandchildren.

As long as the food choices you encourage are for the most part healthy and your child is eating a well-balanced diet, then a few unhealthy treats while spending time with their grandparents will do no long-term harm. If, however, the grandparents provide childcare for your child while you work, it is advisable to sit down and discuss some clear boundaries about providing and encouraging a well-balanced diet.

Using a treat as an incentive

From around 18 months to two years old, you can begin to use the pudding as an incentive for your toddler to finish her meal, if she seems to be struggling with the final spoonfuls of a savoury or main meal. By getting the yoghurt/treat out and showing it to your toddler, you can encourage her to finish the last of her meal. I usually say, 'Look what Mummy has. You eat this last bit and then you can have your yoghurt/treat.' Don't be surprised if the initial reply you are met with is 'No' as your toddler makes a grab for the treat. Be consistent!

If she pushes her plate away refusing to eat any more, then you should say, 'Okay, if you are too full to eat your lunch/tea then there's no yoghurt/treat and Mummy will put it away.' Begin to put it away. If she has a reaction and asks for the treat back, then repeat the instruction: 'Oh, would you like the yoghurt?' The answer is likely to be yes in some way. Repeat 'Okay, well you eat your lunch/tea and then you can have it.'

Maybe offer to help her if she is getting tired and give her lots of praise and encouragement: 'Would you like Mummy to feed you? Let's count the spoonfuls as you eat them, 1, 2.' Let her hold the treat if she wants to, as that will help her feel a little closer to getting it, but do not let her open it or eat it until she has finished the rest of her meal. Give lots of praise when she eats the final spoonful. 'Look, this is the last one and then you can have your yoghurt/treat.' As she eats it, praise her again: 'Good girl, hooray!' High five and clap! Repeat, 'Well done. You ate *all* your lunch/tea and now you can have your treat.'

> **TIP**
>
> I've always found positive verbal praise is enough. I've never needed to use a star or sticker chart for mealtimes — I think that makes too much of a big deal of it, and the idea is not to get into a battle and make mealtimes a pressured situation.

If the mealtime becomes difficult and your toddler is refusing to eat any more whatever you do, then don't battle with her. Just say, 'Okay, you don't want any more?' If she answers 'No' or shakes her head, put the yoghurt or treat away and say, 'Mummy will put the yoghurt/treat away and maybe you can have it later after tea. Let's go and wash your hands and face and get you all cleaned up now you have finished.' I'm sure there are times when you feel too full to eat pudding, so there will also be times when your toddler will feel the same.

Once you leave the table, don't dwell on the fact that your toddler didn't finish her meal. Move straight on to an activity she enjoys to distract her and make her forget about the mealtime.

As long as you are consistent at every mealtime, then you won't have problems with fussiness, tantrums, refusal to eat and demands for sweet foods rather than savoury. Leaving the choice open to your toddler means you don't need to battle and your consistency will stop any pressure during mealtimes. Your toddler will eat when she is hungry – if she only wants half a meal at times, then as long as you don't give a sweet treat she is likely to make up for the smaller meal and eat better on the next occasion you offer food. She will gradually learn what she needs to do to earn the treat.

What is a balanced diet?

A balanced diet provides your toddler with a variety of foods from the five main food groups on a daily basis:

- **Fruit and vegetables:** Aim to give your toddler at least five portions of fruit and vegetables per day. They don't have to be fresh or eaten on their own to count as a portion. You can count the vegetables included as part of a meal or dish you are serving. For example, spaghetti bolognese that contains passata as the tomato sauce and onions and mushrooms would be three portions. Frozen and canned fruit and vegetables also count, as do unsweetened 100 per cent fruit or vegetable juice drinks. Different fruits and vegetables contain different vitamins and minerals so it's important to offer a variety. Some children prefer to eat raw vegetables, and you can use healthy dips such as houmous to encourage them to eat more. Try mashing vegetables such as carrots and swede into potato and adding a little grated cheese if you are having trouble getting your toddler to eat them separately.

- **Starchy foods** such as potatoes, bread, rice or pasta and even breakfast cereals provide energy, nutrients and some fibre. It's advisable to use wholegrain varieties when you can and encourage your toddler to eat potatoes with the skin on if possible. Starch is the most common form of carbohydrates that your toddler needs in her diet. Encouraging your toddler to eat a good breakfast will help to give her energy to start the day. Try to stick to healthy cereals that are unsweetened, vitamin fortified and low in salt, such as Ready Brek, Weetabix, Corn Flakes and Rice Krispies. Porridge is also a good choice, although only instant porridge is fortified with vitamins – you can also add fruit to certain cereals to make them more interesting.

- **Milk and dairy products:** Whole milk and full-fat dairy products are a good source of calcium, which is needed to help your toddler develop strong bones and teeth. They also contain vitamin A, which is needed for healthy skin and eyes and to help the body fight off and resist infections. From the age of 12 months you can give your child cow's milk instead of formula milk, or you may choose to continue breastfeeding. Full-fat milk should be given between the ages of 1–2 years and from the age of two, you can switch to semi-skimmed milk, as long as your toddler eats well and is growing well for her age. Skimmed or 1 per cent fat milk is not recommended for children under the age of five. Try to give your child three servings of milk per day, either as a drink or in foods made from milk, such as cheese, yoghurts, custard and white sauce. Don't be tempted to give too much milk to drink, though, as it can affect appetite and how well the body absorbs nutrients. It can also cause constipation.

- **Non-dairy sources of protein:** Foods such as eggs, beans, meat and fish are a great way to ensure your toddler has enough protein in her diet. You should aim for one or two portions per day. Oily fish such as tuna, salmon, mackerel or sardines should be limited to four portions per week for boys and two portions per week for girls, who may go on to have a baby of their own one day. Oily fish can contain a low level of pollutant that builds up in the body if given too often. For girls, it can affect the development, during pregnancy, of any baby they go on to have. As long as you don't give oily fish too frequently and stick to the recommendations, then the benefits far outweigh the risk.

- Iron is essential for your child's physical and mental development. It can firstly be found in meat and fish and is easily absorbed by the body. Even a small amount of meat or fish is good because it helps the body absorb iron from other food sources. Iron is also found in plant foods but is not so easy for the body to absorb from those, so if your toddler does not eat meat or fish, you need to ensure they eat plenty of dried fruit, dark green leafy vegetables, lentils and fortified breakfast cereals.

- **Foods containing fat, sugar and salt:** Providing your child is a good eater and growing well, you can gradually begin to introduce lower-fat dairy products from the age of two and cut down on fat in other foods. By the time your child is five, she can be eating a healthy low-fat diet that is recommended for adults. In particular, you should keep an eye on the amount of trans-fats in the food your family eats and keep it to a minimum. To reduce fat in meals:

* Use as little oil as possible and choose one that is high in mono- or polyunsaturates like olive, soya or rapeseed. In the UK, pure vegetable oil is often rapeseed oil.
* Remove the skin from poultry.
* Reduce the amount of meat you add to stews and bulk it out with more vegetables and lentils.
* Buy low-fat meat products and lean cuts of meat.
* When cooking or browning mince, drain the fat off before you add gravy or a sauce and continue cooking.
* Grill or bake foods rather than frying them.

Limit the amount of sugar your child has to protect her teeth. The longer and more often sugar touches the teeth, the more damage it does. Brush your toddler's teeth at least once per day but twice if you can. If you give sugary drinks and foods, preferably give them with meals and not as snacks. Water is the best drink to encourage but if your toddler won't drink it give a small amount of juice diluted with water. Never allow your toddler to drink juice from a bottle as this causes great damage to teeth. Always use an open cup for juice or a beaker of water can be offered if your toddler is still trying to master the art of drinking from a cup with no lid.

Salt should not be added to foods that your toddler will be eating, as most foods already contain it and too much can contribute towards high blood pressure later in life. The maximum daily amount of salt for children aged 1–3 years is 2 g and for children aged 4–6 years it is 3 g.

Meal ideas and how to get your toddler to eat healthily

You are your toddler's biggest role model, so it's important that she sees you eating well and making healthy food choices.

The way you present the food to your toddler can make all the difference as to whether she becomes enthusiastic about eating it. One idea is to use a sectioned plate to separate the different food groups. Make a funny shape or face using the items you have put on the plate. If your child can be encouraged to eat the 'eyes, nose and ears' first, before you know it, the plate will be empty with no fuss or cajoling.

Breakfast ideas
- Toast with fruit pieces
- Boiled egg with toasted soldiers
- Cereals fortified with vitamins
- Plain yoghurt with pureed fruit mixed in
- Omelette

Lunch ideas
- Baked beans/cheese/egg on toast
- Pitta with houmous and cucumber, celery and carrot sticks
- Tuna and cucumber sandwich

Supper ideas
- Shepherds pie with vegetables
- Lamb or chicken casserole
- Fish in a white sauce with cheesy vegetables
- Rice, chicken and vegetables

Annabel Karmel (see page 307) has some great cookbooks that you can buy with very simple and easy-to-make recipes that children love and can be eaten by all of the family. I used her books constantly when my children were babies and toddlers and found them a great resource.

Snacks

- Fresh fruit
- Raw vegetables with houmous
- Raisins, sultanas and other dried fruit
- Plain, unsweetened yoghurt
- Canned fruit in fruit juice
- Unsalted rice cakes
- Breadsticks with houmous
- Pitta bread and cheese chunks

If your child is a fussy eater or has a very small appetite, avoid giving snacks between meals. Encourage the habit that she gets to choose a snack after her main meal is finished.

Over-eating and obesity

If a child is carrying excess weight or even obese, the cause is usually over-eating (eating too much of the wrong food types) and under-exercising (not moving around enough). Children learn by example in everything they do, so it's very important to be a good role model. If you want to teach your child to eat healthily and be active, you need to be doing the same yourself. If your child does seem to be putting on excess weight, speak to your GP or health visitor about your concerns, who will weigh your toddler and advise you accordingly.

Transitioning to a sippy cup

For the most part when to make the transition to a sippy cup seems to be a personal choice for individual parents and toddlers. Most health professionals recommend transitioning from a bottle to a sippy cup at around 12 months old, or by two years old at the latest. Some toddlers will happily make this transiton and be ready for it at that age, but many will not. The transition may be influenced by you going back to work and needing your baby or toddler to begin drinking milk from a cup rather than the breast, if she has been breastfeeding. It may also be a natural progression from the bottle/breast to a cup as your baby turns into a toddler.

All three of my children were breastfed but happily accepted a bottle when offered for the first six months. When they were six months I stopped breastfeeding and they went on to formula in a bottle for all of their milk feeds. At 12 months they were all having two bottles per day, one in the morning when they woke and one in the evening before they went to bed. I began giving cow's milk instead of formula at 12 months.

I continued this routine until they were all two years old, at which point I began giving them their morning cow's milk in a sippy cup with their breakfast. I had tried to make the transition slightly earlier with all of them, but they were not very happy at all and as they were only having milk twice a day and not walking around with a bottle constantly for comfort, my personal decision was to allow them to continue with the bottle for a little longer. None of them were very impressed with the idea of losing the bottle even at two years old, and would refuse to drink from a cup and just eat their breakfast without drinking any milk! As they were older and eating a varied diet and getting their calcium intake from various other foods too, I didn't let it worry me and stayed very relaxed even when they refused to touch the milk at all. After a week or two they all began to take small sips of the milk in the mornings and I continued until they were drinking most of it before I decided to change the evening bottle to a sippy cup too! Again, it took a few days of perseverance – my youngest was particularly determined: 'Not cup, Mummy, bottle!' Perseverance paid off again and after showing her that there were no bottles in the cupboard because I had given them to all the little babies, she stopped asking.

As your toddler gets older and more independent, you can progress to allowing her to drink with the lid off the cup or buy one of the special toddler cups that teach and encourage children from a young age how to use a cup without use of the lid. As with anything where babies and toddlers are concerned, patience and perseverance is the key.

Family mealtimes

Where possible, mealtimes should be a family occasion or at least a Mummy (or Daddy) and a toddler experience, right from preparing the food to cook, to serving it and then actually sitting down to eat it. Toddlers love to be involved and help, so give your little one small tasks to do as you are preparing the meal, such as putting the vegetables in the pans as you prepare them and mixing things, for example when you are making a cake. You can encourage her to set the table, with help from you if needed, and help you serve the food too. She will feel more relaxed and want to eat if she sees that you are also having your lunch or tea and she can mimic you. This is also a good way to encourage table manners (see page 57). Try to make sure you are all eating the same foods as often as possible, so you are being the best role model you can be when it comes to eating vegetables and a variety of foods.

Distraction

Chatting to your toddler as you are sitting together eating will provide a good distraction and make mealtimes an enjoyable experience rather than a chore, or a time she dreads because she feels pressured to eat. This is particularly important for children with smaller appetites or fussy eaters.

My two boys always had huge appetites as babies. This was made even more apparent to me once I began to wean my youngest child. She has always had a much smaller appetite compared to her older brothers when they were the same age, and it has taken various distraction tactics to encourage good eating habits. When she was a baby I would give her a spoon to hold and allow her to play with various toys and items as I spoon-fed her. I even sang songs to her towards the end of a meal, once the toys became discarded in a pile on the floor around the highchair, to encourage her to eat the last few spoonfuls. Not surprisingly she never needed any encouragement to eat her pudding or sweet treat afterwards!

Her appetite remains small to this day. However, it has been easier to encourage good eating habits once she began to understand about choice and the consequences of her choices. I am now able to give her the option of a nice pudding and if she shows enthusiasm for it, I encourage her to finish her main meal first. She now understands that if she doesn't want to eat a reasonable amount of her first course then there won't be any pudding offered.

Watching TV during the odd mealtime may be something you feel is okay as a treat. As long as it doesn't distract your child from eating, I personally don't see an issue with it every now and then. We always try to have family mealtimes at the table, but if my daughter and I are home alone in the daytime then we love nothing better than snuggling up on the sofa together with our sandwich at lunchtime and watching the TV as we eat.

Table manners

Mealtimes are a good opportunity to teach your child good manners. Eating with her mouth closed and not speaking when she has food in her mouth are both good habits that she can learn by mimicking you. These are habits that you can encourage by just reminding her gently to finish what is in her mouth before speaking or by asking her to watch how you eat with your mouth closed. It is good habits like these that are taught during family mealtimes where you or older siblings can set good examples.

Please and thank you

You can begin to teach your child good manners when she is very young. Please and thank you can be said by you when giving and receiving food, toys and other items from when your child is a small baby. I use the shortened version of 'thank you', 'ta', when giving to or receiving from babies, as it's an easier word for them to use and encourages manners and appreciation from an early age.

When your baby's speech develops as she transitions to becoming a toddler, you can progress to saying 'thank you' or 'please' after also saying 'ta' in the relevant situations. This will encourage her to begin using the grown-up manners that older children and adults endorse, and in my experience the transition is always very natural and smooth. If you do not like or want your baby or toddler to be encouraged to use the shortened version of thank you or please, that is perfectly okay. Just be aware that it will take a little longer for her to grasp the concept of using her manners as you need to wait until she is older and able to actually say the words please and thank you.

Different families have various table manners that they deem acceptable or not. Eating certain foods with their fingers, not putting elbows on the table, and placing cutlery together at the end of the meal are all examples of manners you may want to encourage in your children. You may feel some are more important than others. It is up to you to encourage and teach your child, by example, how to sit and eat her food in an acceptable fashion to you. Just remember not to be too strict to begin with. As she gets older she will naturally want to copy you anyway without you turning mealtimes into a strict, pressured time.

Using cutlery

Although you may have been giving your baby a spoon to hold since you first began weaning, she won't have learnt to do anything other than wave it around menacingly! She will happily chew on it, but to go from that to using it as a means to get food into her mouth takes a great deal of skill.

The choice to be independent and begin to *want* to feed themselves varies between toddlers and depends somewhat on their physical development. Some will be fiercely independent and get very cross if a parent tries to help them. They get equally frustrated when they lack the physical dexterity to use a spoon or fork and the food they do manage to load falls off before it reaches their mouth.

Having lots of opportunity to practise this new skill is the only way your toddler will improve at it. Begin with easier foods, such as pasta, that aren't too difficult to load on to cutlery. You can then move on to more difficult foods, such as custard and jelly, although even adults can struggle to keep jelly on the spoon! If your child is struggling, you may be able to use distraction to sneak the odd spoon or forkful of food into her mouth yourself to ensure she eats something at least, but try to keep the mealtime as relaxed as possible.

It will be normal for your toddler to use a combination of trying the spoon and fork and using her hands to pick the food up. Don't pester her about the way she is doing it at this early stage of learning, or you will put her off trying at all. Her competence at using the cutlery will improve the more she practises.

As independent as some toddlers are, you may have a child who is quite happy being spoon-fed and shows no desire to make the effort to feed herself. She may have tried on the odd occasion and become so frustrated that it wasn't as easy as anticipated, so refused to try again.

Always give her a spoon and fork at mealtimes to encourage independence but don't worry if she doesn't want to try. As with all developmental stages, all children want and learn skills at varying ages, even siblings. When it comes to self-feeding, patience and perseverance are needed in abundance – children all do it in their own time. I'm sure you have never seen a 4- or 5-year-old being totally spoon-fed at every meal!

TIP

Try busying yourself in the kitchen while your child is eating if sitting with her doesn't help. At times your presence at the table will make her feel more pressured. Put her meal in front of her with cutlery and then empty the dishwasher or tidy up. Appear busy but keep an eye on how your toddler is getting on. You may find that she naturally begins trying to feed herself without having you sat there as an audience actively watching her.

Handling the mess!

Mess is an inevitable result of your toddler beginning to learn to feed herself a range of different foods, some of which can be particularly difficult to manoeuvre on to the spoon and into her mouth – jelly and spaghetti are particularly tricky examples. Toddlers like to be independent so they are unlikely to want you to help. Your toddler may get cross and even refuse to eat if you get involved. So it is best to leave her to it and stay relaxed about the mess that is made, so she feels no pressure when eating. You could put a big plastic sheet under the chair where she sits if you want to make the mess on the floor around her easier to clean up afterwards and have a warm flannel or wet wipes to hand after she has finished each meal.

Finger foods

Most babies and toddlers love the idea of finger foods and will happily try most things at least once. As you first began offering finger foods when your toddler was a baby you may have noticed that she had a preference towards certain flavours, items or even textured food.

From an early age some babies really don't like the idea of picking up anything wet and slimy that can break or squish in their hands and make them a bit mucky. They may prefer to hold a solid food instead and refuse to eat any finger foods that they can't get a good grip of. This can continue into toddlerhood and some children really do not like the idea of getting mess on their hands and potentially their clothes too, so will refuse to touch anything that might have that effect.

As long as your toddler is getting a varied diet from the main meals that you feed her, it doesn't matter if she will only hold and feed herself certain finger foods. As long as you are very relaxed about her feeding herself and don't make her nervous about being messy at mealtimes, she will eventually begin to try new things when encouraged.

CASE STUDY: Michelle and Oliver

Oliver had never been that enthusiastic about eating solid food even from the early stages of weaning. In particular, once finger foods were introduced he refused point blank to pick anything up that was wet or slimy and would struggle to process lumpy food as he got older, and vomit if his mother Michelle attempted to offer him any. As he got older the food issues were getting worse instead of better and Michelle was very stressed about his food intake on a daily basis.

Michelle reached out to me via Twitter and asked for advice. I offered her some basic tips and was luckily halfway through writing this food chapter for the toddler book, so offered to send it to her as soon as it was complete. This is her feedback after reading it and using the advice:

'I've tried everything to get Oliver to eat — shouting, ignoring him, technically letting him go hungry, giving in to yoghurt, living off banana, the lot. The only thing that has had consistent results is this method. For about three weeks I've stuck to the chapter and each day had some improvement. But not once did I give him a pudding if he didn't eat dinner and I always acted calm (even if I wanted to cry) and got him out of the highchair without fuss. He's 21 months and not a massive talker but today I said, 'Okay, no dinner, no yoghurt.' He said, 'Okay,' and ate some dinner. He then said, 'Yoghurt?' I said, 'No, dinner first,' and this continued till he finished his dinner and then had his yoghurt! I'm going to stick to this plan and

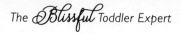

reread the chapter if I ever get lost. It is honestly the only method that has ever worked!'

Michelle continues to use the advice in this chapter and although she has good days and days where Oliver doesn't eat so much, things are much better and he is now trying a variety of foods, finishing his meals when he's hungry enough for pudding and happily eating a range of finger foods too.

Throwing food

Younger toddlers tend to throw food when they are bored of eating or don't want to eat something, or even as a sign they have finished their meal, especially if their language skills are not developed enough to actually express this. Throwing food is a habit you need to nip in the bud as quickly as possible, particularly if you have a dog. It's amazing how quickly toddlers learn to secretly feed the dog when they don't want to eat something.

Try to spot the signs that your toddler is getting bored of whatever food she has on her tray before she starts dropping it over the edge of her chair. If she's playing with her food and not really eating any more, you can ask if she's finished. If you feel she's eaten enough, ask her to pass the remaining food to you or, if able to, put it in the bin herself.

If you don't think she has eaten enough, you can use the pudding tactic (see page 46) to encourage her to eat a little more. If she drops the food on the floor without you managing to stop or distract her first, then pick it up and just gently remind her to pass it to you if she doesn't want any more. For example, say, 'Not on the floor, please. If you don't want it, then give it to Mummy and say, "No more, Mummy".' Say 'No more, Mummy' in a silly voice to make the idea of giving it to you fun. Show her what you want to do by picking up another piece off her tray and passing it to you, saying, 'No more, Mummy.' She will soon get the idea and stop throwing it on the floor if you are consistent

Eating out

You may worry about eating out with your toddler. What will she eat? Will she behave? Will it be too stressful to be enjoyable? Once you have established good eating and table manners at home, it will be much easier to encourage that when you are eating out. Many child-friendly restaurants will be flexible with the menu choices they offer and will take off or add certain food choices to the dish if you just ask. *My husband is always a bit embarrassed when I do it, but if you don't ask, you don't get! The worst they will say is, 'No, sorry, we can't do that,' so I never see any harm in asking. In one restaurant we go to regularly that has 'Pasta in a tomato sauce' on the menu, I ask them to do the pasta with a carbonara sauce instead and add pieces of chicken breast to it, as I know my toddler daughter will much prefer that. They have this option on the adult menu, so I know they have the ingredients, but I don't want to order and pay for an adult portion for a toddler. They have always been very obliging and agreed to my request, despite not actually having that on their children's menu.*

Most restaurants will usually provide colouring and activity books for children while they wait for their meal. If you are not sure if the place you are going to will do that, it's worth taking some from home to keep your toddler busy. We play games such as 'I Spy' too, as keeping your children happy and distracted while waiting for the food to arrive will stop them being tempted to misbehave.

*

Your toddler will learn from you, so it's important that you teach her the right messages regarding eating a healthy diet and how to behave at mealtimes. Encourage her to co-operate at mealtimes and follow the examples you and any older siblings set to make mealtimes a positive and enjoyable experience for all of you.

3
Toddler behaviour

If you haven't read Chapter 1, Sleep Solutions, yet I advise you to do so before reading this chapter. Good sleep is the key to good behaviour. It paves the way for the rest of your toddler's day to run smoothly, from eating well, to being much more open to negotiation when sharing and playing with others. If you sort any sleep issues out, it will be much easier to encourage and teach good behaviour on a day-to-day basis.

We all know how it feels to be sleep deprived. You are unlikely to be in the best of moods the following day if you haven't had a decent night's sleep. When you feel tired, your patience and effort at various activities is likely to wear down very quickly and you will become frustrated or even angry in a much shorter timeframe. Babies, toddlers and older children are no different. If they are tired from not getting a regular and good night's sleep, it is likely to affect their behaviour and make them more difficult to manage.

'The terrible twos'
I have heard this phrase so often to describe toddler behaviour. Many parents worry before their child is aged two, knowing this stage is on its way. It is known as 'the terrible twos' because

between 2–3 years is often the age that parents find hardest in terms of their toddler's behaviour. But in my experience, and from talking to other parents, this 'testing' behaviour may even start as early as 18 months.

As your baby transitions into becoming a toddler, he is learning so much about the environment and people around him. There are many things that he will desperately *want* to do, but he may not yet have developed the physical skills and this will cause him a great deal of frustration. Equally, there may be things he wants that are out of reach, or things that he would like to copy older siblings doing, but without the speech to relay and vocalise what he wants, he will become very frustrated.

It is this frustration that causes what are commonly known as 'temper tantrums'. They are a perfectly normal part of your child's toddler years. It is how you react to them that will determine how often the tantrums happen and how difficult they are to manage.

Distraction

As a parent of a toddler, and having worked as a nanny for many years, I have found that distraction is the best way to prevent or stop a tantrum before it reaches fever pitch! You simply divert your toddler's attention and enable him to forget the activity or problem that was potentially going to cause a tantrum. This technique will be your best friend for the next 2–3 years at least. It still amazes me how easy it is to stop a tantrum in its tracks, just by making something else seem much more interesting.

It is important to acknowledge the potential cause of a tantrum first and then deal with it accordingly, explaining to your toddler why he can't do or have something. Then use your best distraction skills immediately afterwards to prevent your negative answer turning your toddler into a screaming, angry heap on the floor! For example: Your toddler goes into the cupboard and helps himself to some sweets. You don't want him to have them. Remove him from the cupboard, put the treats back and say, 'We are not having treats now as it will soon be lunch/supper time. You can maybe have some afterwards.' If you think he may be hungry but you don't want him having treats, then offer an alternative, such as a piece of fruit. If he refuses and asks for the sweets again, repeat and offer the fruit alternative again. If he doesn't want that, immediately take him out of the kitchen to remove the temptation and make it clear that you are not going to change your mind. As you are walking away with him, say something like, 'Wow, why don't we go and get the trains/dolls/bricks, etc., to play with?' Engage him in an activity that you know he usually loves – make it sound very exciting and much more interesting than what you left behind.

If your toddler continues to thrash around in your arms and protest about not getting what he wants, let him. Lie him down on the floor somewhere safe and then begin to play with some of his toys by yourself, talking loudly and enthusiastically and sounding really interested in what you are doing. Try to engage him by asking him to help or encouraging him to show you how to do something – pretend that you can't do it yourself. He will soon get bored of rolling around on the floor making lots of noise if he gets no direct attention for it and you don't give in to his initial demand in the first place.

If you have a very strong-willed toddler and your attempts at trying to distract him with a new activity *still* don't work, then I would suggest you leave the room completely. Ensure he is in a safe room and environment and say to him as you are leaving the room, 'Mummy is going to go into the other room as all that noise you are making is making my head hurt. When you stop that noise, we can have a cuddle and play with some toys together.' Walk out of the room and wait for 30–60 seconds. Return to the room and say something like, 'Have you finished making that noise yet? Shall we have a cuddle and find some toys to play with?' If he continues, then leave again and say, 'No, you are not finished? Okay, I will go away again.' Keep returning at 30–60-second intervals until he is ready to listen and calm down.

You can also use your toddler's bedroom as a safe place to put him to calm down, particularly if you are upstairs. Ideally, you will have a stair gate on the doorframe so that he can't run straight back out of the room. To ensure this doesn't have a negative effect on his bedtime routine and settling, make sure you are clear that your toddler is going into the room to calm down or for time out and not being put to bed as any kind of punishment.

Keep returning to the room. Once your toddler is ready to listen and stops crying, have a nice cuddle together and praise him for stopping the noise. Ask him what he would like to go and find to play with together. Turn the whole thing into something nice you do together as a reward for him stopping the tantrum.

It is important to acknowledge your toddler's feelings of frustration at not getting what he wants, without rewarding his cries with the thing that he has been told he can't have. It's normal for him to be angry that things haven't gone his way. By giving him the time and space to let his frustration out, you are able to respect and acknowledge his feelings without giving in to him all the time.

If your toddler is still developing his language skills he may cry in frustration. Encourage him to use the words he does have or show you. I've always said, 'No crying. Use your words and show me and I will help you.' Kneel down so you are at eye level with him and ask him questions, such as 'Do you need me to help you? What do you want me to do?' Once you know what he wants, you can then decide whether it's a request you are happy to grant! If you encourage him more towards talking and showing you the reasons for his frustrations, he will gradually learn to do that naturally without the need for getting cross regularly.

With an older toddler who is three or four years old, you will be able to explain and chat about frustrations more easily: 'I know you are cross because you want to have the sweeties now, but we have to have lunch first. If you eat nicely, then maybe you can have some afterwards. Okay?'

> ### TIP
>
> *As parents you both need to be 'singing from the same song sheet'. Don't let your toddler play you off against each other. If he knows that when Mummy says no, Daddy will say yes, then overall you lose a little bit of control, and his respect for you and the things you say will diminish. It is likely to cause ongoing behaviour issues, particularly for the parent who is being regularly undermined.*

Negotiation and choice

Lots of things may frustrate your toddler on a day-to-day basis, but if he feels like he has a little bit of choice and decision-making in most activities, he will happily go with the flow without the need for any major meltdowns! Negotiation and choice are powerful parenting tools you can use to encourage your toddler to do certain things.

Allow him to develop his independence by offering him choices on a daily basis. This will help him feel a little more in control of his daily activities, even though technically you still have full control. Stick to a simple choice between two things – don't complicate it by offering too many options.

Learn to pick your battles

Getting dressed can sometimes be a battle. Toddlers have a very odd dress sense at times and their request to wear a pair of shorts and a vest top when it's freezing cold outside isn't one you can agree to! However, you can still offer choice by allowing your toddler to choose between two acceptable pairs of trousers that would be warm enough and two acceptable tops. Ask him to decide between the two outfits on offer. You can compromise with his choice of outfit by saying he can wear shorts in the house, but when it is time to go out then he needs to put warmer clothes on like Mummy.

TIP

You can reduce the risk of a heated debate over outfits in the first place by being organised each morning and giving your toddler two just options of clothing to choose from, before he has the chance to root around in his things.

My three-year-old daughter was dressed in a lovely black-and-white dress recently, with her hair done to match in nice bobbles and a flower, all ready to go out. When I gave her the matching black shoes to wear she kicked up a fuss and told me she didn't want to wear them. She wanted to wear her scuffed pink ones that lit up, the ones we usually save for pre-school. We were going somewhere nice for lunch so I wasn't prepared to allow her to wear the pink ones that wouldn't match. However, we still had 20 minutes before we needed to leave, so I told her she could wear the pink ones with her dress for a little while until it was time to go and she would then have to change into the black ones. She was quite happy with this compromise and when it was time to go, she happily changed into the black shoes with the promise that she could put the pink ones back on when we returned home – everyone was happy and a potential tantrum was avoided!

With food you can offer your toddler a choice of pudding, for example raisins or banana. Again, giving him a choice makes him feel more independent and like he has some control in his life.

Don't battle with your toddler and turn things into a 'Yes you will, no you won't' argument. If you offer a choice about clothes, in particular, and he doesn't want to listen, walk away. Say something like, 'Well, you are making me a bit sad as you are not listening to me. I'm going to walk away and come back when you have decided which outfit you want to wear because we can't go out until we are both dressed.' Trust me, if you are not standing there battling with him, then he will soon come round to your way of thinking!

> **TIP**
>
> *Toddlers really don't like to be rushed, so always try to allow enough time to give them a choice and time to encourage them to do things willingly after explanations from you.*

I always find toddlers will be much more inclined to listen if you give them a reason for whatever you want them to do. They like to know what is going on and why. Again it falls back to making them feel in control of situations in order to develop their independence and understand the world around them. Respect works both ways. If you want your toddler to respect you and listen to you, he has to, in turn, feel like he is listened to and has a degree of choice on a day-to-day basis. That doesn't mean allowing him to do what he wants whenever he wants – all that will achieve is making him spoilt and continuing to always expect you to back down and give in to him.

Explain to him the reasons for doing things. For example:

- 'Right, it's time to put our coat and shoes on as we have to collect your brothers from school.'
- 'We need to close the door because the dog will run outside if you don't.'
- 'I know you want to pour the drink yourself, but it is very heavy, so I might need to help you a little bit, otherwise it will go everywhere.'

Give your toddler the instruction and the reason for it. Encourage him to follow it through and give lots of praise when he does. You should then use your best distraction methods to talk about different things or an activity you did earlier or plan to do, so that he's diverted away from any potential meltdown.

When there just isn't time

There will, of course, be days when despite your best intentions you have to rush around as you may be running late for something. Your patience for explaining things may not be on top form as you rush your toddler into his shoes and coat to get out of the house quickly. It is inevitable that he is likely to be as fractious and stressed as you at being rushed out the door.

I would bet money on the fact that every parent of a toddler has been short-tempered with their child at least once in their life, particularly when rushing or running late for something. The important thing is to acknowledge it and actually apologise to your toddler if you think you have been unreasonable – after all, that is what you would expect from him if you didn't like his behaviour. Say to him something like, 'I'm sorry I shouted at you to hurry up and get your coat and shoes on. I was just worried we were going to be late but I shouldn't have shouted at you. Can we have a big cuddle together?'

If your toddler sees and hears that you apologise when you are in the wrong, it will be much easier to encourage him to do the same if he upsets you or one of his friends. He will see apologising and trying to make someone feel happy again a normal thing to do. Children learn by example – if you show him the correct way to act, he will naturally follow suit.

Teaching your toddler to apologise

Toddlers very quickly learn that certain actions and behaviour won't get a great reaction. A young toddler can be encouraged to give an 'apology cuddle', or even just a handshake, if he hurts someone else. Your reaction will show your toddler the way to behave so, for example, if he does hurt you he will see that he has made you sad. You can encourage him to give you an apology cuddle and then put a big smiley face on afterwards – this way he sees the different reactions and enjoys the positive one. As his speech and language develops, he can be encouraged to use the word 'sorry' if he hurts someone/something. If you practise these skills at home and also give him the respect back, by apologising to him when you are also in the wrong, as described above, then he will soon understand what is expected of him.

What is 'naughty behaviour'?

One of the biggest things that was drummed into all of us as students when we did our nursery nurse training was that there is *naughty behaviour* but not naughty children – and it has stuck in my head ever since! It is *very* important to label the behaviour and what a child is doing as naughty or silly, rather than labelling the child – by doing this and dealing with the unwanted behaviour in the correct way, you will have a much lower chance of repeated and regular occurrences.

For example, if your toddler hits you, *don't* say, 'You are a very naughty boy – hitting isn't nice!' Instead say, 'Hitting was a very naughty thing to do. You have made me sad now. Can I have a cuddle to make me feel better and can you say sorry for hurting me please?' Don't say '*You* are silly', but instead say '*It's* a very silly thing to do and *it's* making me sad. Please can you stop it now!'

As long as your voice is firm enough when telling your toddler off he will understand that he has upset you with behaviour you don't like. I personally am not keen on the word naughty at all. I have always found referencing certain aspects of behaviour as 'silly' a much better option. For example: 'Please don't do that – it is very silly. Let's go and find some nice toys to play with instead.' I would save the word 'naughty' for an act that has been done deliberately – most likely something your toddler knows that you really wouldn't want him to do, but chooses to do anyway – for example, throwing a toy across the room in frustration, or hurting another person.

Your tone of voice when one of the more serious actions occurs should also be clear, again with no need for shouting, but a deep enough tone and a stern enough look on your face to let your toddler know that you are very unhappy with that type of behaviour. Encourage him to pick up the toy he has thrown or apologise to whoever he has hurt, after explaining why he shouldn't have done it. Explaining why he shouldn't do something will help him understand and learn from it for the future. For example:

- 'We don't throw things because they might break. You and Mummy and Daddy will be very sad if we can't play with it any more and have to put it into the bin.'
- 'We don't hit or hurt people because it makes them cry and say "Ow!" You need to cuddle your friend and say sorry to make him happy again.'

When your toddler does what you ask to correct his behaviour, use big positive gestures, such as a really happy face, a big cuddle and lots of praise. Tell him what a clever and good boy he is for listening to you. Toddlers want to please and make people happy. They very quickly learn the difference between happy and sad. If your toddler realises that certain actions and behaviour make you sad, he can be encouraged to make you happy again by apologising and changing his behaviour. He will enjoy the rewards of affection and praise that follow.

Alternatively, if he refuses to pick up the toy or apologise straight away because he is still cross, a little bit of 'time out' is probably needed.

Time out

We all get frustrated at times and toddlers are no different. As an adult we recognise when we are cross and, when possible, we walk away from a situation to calm down and clear our head. When we return, we are less likely to get angry. Your toddler will not have the ability to recognise when he needs time out to calm down and talk to you more reasonably, so he needs you to implement that at times, especially when he's younger.

If you have tried to reason with your toddler by giving him choices, and have used your best distraction skills to try to prevent a tantrum, but it comes anyway, then you need to give him a time and place to calm down.

If I'm at home and downstairs, then I tend to use 'the silly step' for my children. I've heard lots of people call it 'the naughty step' but as I mentioned previously, I don't like to use that word very often. So in our house, since I used it for the first time with my eldest son 11 years ago, it has always been known as 'the silly step'.

I advise parents to use the warning method that I used with my own three children, and the children I looked after when working as a nanny. First you say, 'If you do that again or don't listen to me, then I'm going to put you on the silly step.'

Let's take throwing a toy as an example: Your toddler throws a toy across the room in frustration. You say, 'Don't throw things, please. It might hit someone or break. We play with toys nicely. Can you go and pick it up, please?' Hopefully your toddler will listen and go to retrieve it. If he does, praise him and then immediately distract him with another toy or activity. You have let him know that you don't want him to do something and why, and then distracted him with something more positive.

If he refuses to pick the toy up when asked, or he throws something else, then you should say something like: 'Mummy said not to throw things, didn't I? I want you to go and pick it up now. If you don't, or you throw anything else, then I'm going to sit you on the silly step for not listening to me.'

If he throws something else or refuses to pick up the thrown toy, then he is definitely testing the boundaries to see if you will actively follow through. Leave the thrown toy on the floor and pick him up or walk him to the stairs and say something like, 'You need to sit here on the silly step because you didn't listen to Mummy and were throwing toys and not picking them up when I asked you to.'

Sit him on the bottom step (or the second or third step if you have a stair gate at the bottom of the stairs like us). As you sit him there, you should say something like: 'Mummy is sitting you on the silly step because you were throwing things. I asked you to stop and you didn't listen and now Mummy is sad. You need to stay there until I come to get you.'

I recommend you use one minute of time per year of life, so if your toddler is two years old then time out is for two minutes, at three years old it is three minutes, etc. It's quite helpful to use a beeper as your toddler gets older. Most ovens have a timer that will beep once it has counted down. This is good for your toddler to listen out for and he knows that means it's the end of his time out and you will come back. Alternatively, you could use a sand timer that you make yourself and turn upside down, leaving it visible to your toddler but out of reach. You could also use a basic egg timer.

When you first begin to use the silly step, I think it is better not to use a timer at all. Even a 20–30-second time out on the silly step will usually be enough for your toddler to re-think his behaviour and want to get off the stairs and do what you originally asked to make you happy again.

The silly step can begin to be used with some 18-month-olds who have good understanding and language already. It's not always about getting children to say sorry for their actions – that will come later, as they get older. The important thing is that you let your toddler know that his actions are unacceptable and in the case of throwing a toy, encourage him to rectify his behaviour by picking the toy up and putting it away nicely.

I would suggest walking away, counting to 20–30, then going back to him and saying, 'Right, are you going to come and play nicely now without throwing things?' If he says yes then say, 'Okay, you need to say sorry to Mummy for not listening and I want you to go and pick the toy up that you were throwing and put it away again.' Hopefully you should get a 'Sorry Mummy' and then you can have a nice cuddle. Remind your toddler as he gets off the silly step that if he throws anything else, he will have to come back to the silly step again. Encourage him to pick up the thrown toy, praise him and then move on by distracting him with a new activity.

If he gets off the step as soon as you have put him on it, which is very likely the first few times you implement this method, just keep placing him there again saying, 'Stay there until Mummy comes to get you.' If he really won't stay and continues to get off then say, 'Okay, are you going to come and play nicely now? Come and pick up the toy for Mummy, please, and put it back and then we can play with something else.' By still following through with letting him know he wasn't behaving well and encouraging him to pick up the thrown toy, the very short time out he had will be enough to encourage more positive behaviour. Give him lots of praise when he picks the toy up and then distract him with another activity.

If he has stayed on the step as directed but is not ready to say sorry after the first 20–30 seconds, say something like, 'You are not ready? Okay, Mummy will go away and come back again soon.' Go away and return in another 20–30 seconds and ask again. It will only take a few times of using the silly step for your toddler to realise and understand when he has to go there.

My youngest daughter, who has just turned three years old, will sometimes say 'Yes' when I ask her if she wants me to put her on the silly step! I call her bluff and do it and walk away and she will then call me and say, 'Mum, I'm not being silly now. Can I get off now, please?' When I go back she is suddenly much more reasonable!

If you are upstairs and you want to use your toddler's bedroom as the place for the time out, you can do that as an alternative. As long as you don't use his actual bed, it should not have a negative impact or become associated with bedtime and sleep, as some health professionals or experts may suggest. Time out is not about shutting your toddler away, shouting or getting cross. It is about giving your toddler a safe and quiet place to calm down so that you can reason with him again. It also gives you the opportunity to calm down if his behaviour is being particularly trying and testing your patience.

When you are away from home or at a friend's house, or even if you live in a flat or bungalow that doesn't have stairs, you can improvise a 'silly spot or corner'. Choose an area of the house that is your silly spot. You could even buy a small coloured doormat or rug that you leave in that area all the time, so that you, your partner and toddler all know where the area is. If you are visiting a friend, then simply move your toddler to a different safe environment – you are giving him time out of the room where the unwanted behaviour is occurring.

Fun parenting

Although you need to have boundaries and rules as parents, to keep your children safe and teach them right from wrong, you also need to enjoy them and have fun together. Happy children who are getting lots of attention will generally behave themselves. Children thrive on the attention of others and enjoy having people around them. If they understand that silly behaviour from them causes a negative response and makes you sad, they won't want that reaction. However, if you are busy and unable to give your child attention, it is highly likely he will do something silly in order to *get* your attention. For a child, any attention is always better than no attention at all.

There is usually always a trigger or reason for your toddler to begin misbehaving. If you can prevent or divert the reason for it and distract him towards doing something positive then the silly behaviour will stop.

Outings

The excitement of being away from the home environment is bound to affect your toddler's listening skills – they are unlikely to be at their best! Use that excitement to your advantage if your toddler is tempted to run off. 'Quick, let's go this way and find the ...' When out shopping use your toddler's enthusiasm to help you and encourage independence by giving him jobs in the supermarket or shop, such as, 'I need you to help me find the apples.'

Count things, talk about any colours you can see. Outings are an amazing teaching experience for your toddler to learn about the world around him. He will be excited by so much of it, so encourage it rather than give negative reactions – your outings or shopping trips will be a much nicer experience for both of you.

While out and about with my own children, I hear and see so many other parents with their toddlers and older children. The relaxed, calm parents are having a much happier time allowing their children to wander and explore in front of them, not too far of course, but at least enjoying a little freedom. The parents who sound stressed seem to be the ones trying to keep their children holding their hands and not allowing them any freedom at all to gently explore their surroundings, with that happy excitement and enthusiasm only small children possess!

Give your toddler a little freedom – don't be too strict. Excitement in a new environment will naturally cause some silly behaviour. Children respond better if they're having fun and it's usually easy to encourage them to do the right things with distraction techniques. In short, relax a little. If you are relaxed then your toddler will also be much less likely to misbehave and he will respond better to any directions or instructions you give to him.

Consistency and boundaries

Being a parent is tough, particularly once your baby transitions to a toddler and your patience is being tested daily. He's learning about the world around him, has lots of developmental and environmental changes happening – toilet training, beginning pre-school or nursery, possibly having a new sibling – so it is very normal for him to push boundaries occasionally. He has to work out what he is or isn't allowed to do with various child carers and may even find that Daddy lets him do things that Mummy doesn't, and vice versa, when in the care of only one parent (see page 69).

As parents we all have different patience thresholds in comparison to our friends and their children. We also all have different standards of acceptable behaviour that we allow from our children. As long as your toddler is aware of *your* rules and boundaries and you stick to them, he will feel secure and reassured by your consistency. You may occasionally get comments, such as, 'Jane is having sweeties, can I have some please?'

If you decide that your answer is no then don't back down and give in to social pressure. If you do, your toddler will remember that and be determined to persevere with asking you repeatedly next time, until you give in again.

If you feel pressure to let your child do something he wouldn't normally do in a social situation, because others are, then it is better to say yes as soon as you are asked, rather than as a result of continued pressure. For example, in the case of asking for sweets, let him know it is a special treat: 'Okay, Mummy will let you have the sweets as we are on a special outing, but usually we have sweets *after* lunch don't we?' That small reminder will reinforce your usual rules and mean that you're making the decision rather than being pressured by your toddler.

Praise and rewards

Praising your toddler and letting him see how happy his actions and words make you will always reinforce and encourage good behaviour. Toddlers love to be told they are doing a great job or are clever or very good at something. If you concentrate on the positives, then your toddler's confidence will build daily, which in turn will improve his independence.

I have always tended to use over-the-top praise for good behaviour, helpfulness and kind gestures. Examples include:

- 'Wow, you are so good at tidying! That is making me very happy. Give me a high five!'
- 'Look at your plate – you ate *all* your supper. High five me!'

In case you haven't heard of it 'high five' is where you raise your hand and hit your palms together. Another positive way to praise is by clapping your hands and saying 'Hooray' in a really over-the-top way when your toddler does something you ask, finishes something or does something well. He will love the excitement in your face and voice and immediately want to do something else similar to get the same reaction. The 'hooray' praise is particularly useful when teaching your toddler new things. *I use it for colour or counting activities and my daughter gets so excited by the praise that she is keen to repeatedly do the activity. As you are probably aware, repetition is key to helping a child to learn something. You have most likely heard the phrase 'practice makes perfect'. For example, I will begin a counting activity with her and say, 'Mummy first 1, 2, 3, 4, 5,' and do it in a sing-song voice, then ask her to copy me. Each time she gets it right I shout, 'Hooray!' and clap my hands really excitedly with a big smile on my face. If she gets it wrong, I keep things very relaxed and say, 'No silly, it's 1, 2, 3, 4, 5,' in a silly voice again.*

My daughter thinks it is funny to say 'silly me' when she does get things wrong. She will also say it if she drops something or knocks something over. Accidents happen, of course, and if you save your firm voice for the battles that you really need to have, your child will be much more likely to listen and respond to you. My toddler also says 'silly Mummy' or 'silly Daddy' if we drop something or do something silly as that is what we have taught her.

Behaviour is learned and if your toddler knows that sometimes adults also get things wrong and act in a silly way, it will help his whole understanding of there being a time and place for funny, silly behaviour and also actions that are never acceptable.

Using rewards/sticker charts

Reward/sticker charts are a great tool for transition changes when distraction and verbal rewards don't seem to be enough. Try using them for:

- **Sleep issues:** Transitioning from the cot to bed and encouraging your toddler to stay in bed rather than getting out frequently (see pages 17–24).

- **Toilet training:** As a reward for going on the potty or toilet (see pages 163–78).
- **Sharing and general good behaviour:** If this is something your toddler is struggling with.
- **A new sibling arriving:** As a reward for kind and good behaviour.

You can buy reward charts from various shops, but I find it is better to create my own. It is easier to personalise a home-made one with the targets and areas you want to concentrate on for your individual child. Buy some special stickers that you know your toddler will love – maybe stickers of a TV or book character that he's particularly keen on. He will then be much more enthusiastic and willing to try and do things in order to earn his special stickers.

It is also good to offer a reward once your toddler has earned a certain number of stickers so that he has an extra incentive and treat to work towards and look forward to. For example, three stickers equal a trip to the park and five stickers equal a different treat or outing that you know he will love.

Button/penny jar

An alternative for a child who isn't really interested in stickers or reward charts is having a special button or penny jar for good behaviour. You can buy various coloured and shaped buttons for your toddler to choose from each time he does something great to earn a button. Talking about the colours and shapes can also provide a distraction and become a positive learning experience too.

Some toddlers absolutely love the idea of having money and trying to earn it, just as they see and begin to understand we as

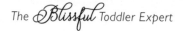

adults have to. It is a good lesson to teach your children from an early age and offering them small change, such as 1p and 2p coins, can be a fantastic incentive for them to listen and do nice things. Not everyone will agree with the idea of using pennies as a reward in a jar, but if you have a toddler who is particularly intrigued and interested in coins, I personally don't see the harm in using it to your advantage. Your toddler may not understand the exact value of that money, but teaching him the basic example that hard work and effort is rewarded and he can then go and spend that reward at the shop, is always going to be a valuable lesson to learn for future use!

Sharing

Most babies develop into selfish toddlers who want and need everything their own way. This is normal. As parents, we have the huge responsibility of turning our little whirlwinds into caring, sharing, patient little people.

A lot of toddler behaviour is learned and can be corrected by providing a happy, stimulating environment that shows the correct way to behave in a firm but equally caring manner.

If your toddler sees you sharing and being kind and gentle with others, it will go a long way to encouraging and teaching that same behaviour in him. Although it is very normal for him to be a grab-and-run type of toddler when he sees a toy he wants, your reaction to his actions will teach him the correct way to behave. Rather than steaming in, shouting 'No' at him and embarrassingly pulling him away, as you hand the toy back to the other toddler and escape red-faced away from the other parent, try a different approach. He needs to understand the consequences and results that his actions cause in order to learn not to do them again. If there is a reason not to do something, then it makes it much easier for a toddler to comprehend. If you drag him away, how can he understand what he did wrong? He saw a toy, wanted it and went to get it. That's what he would do at home, but of course he has to be taught to behave slightly differently in social situations and to wait his turn. Use the happy/sad descriptions for his actions as described earlier on pages 74–6.

My approach would be to go over and say, 'Billy was playing with that toy wasn't he? Now he's sad because you took it away from him. Can you give it back to him please to make him happy again and we will go and find another toy?' Encourage him to hand it over, praise him for doing so and apologise on behalf of him, as it is unlikely he will have the words or understanding to know what he is apologising for to begin with. You should then distract his attention towards an alternative toy or activity that you need to make sound much more exciting!

As your toddler gets older and understands that his actions can cause upset, you can encourage him to say sorry for his behaviour. Explain to him that he can have the toy when the other child has finished, and try to make a point of allowing him a turn with it as a reward for his patience. If, for example, Billy is taking a while to finish playing with the toy and your toddler is getting impatient, keep praising him and reminding him he has to wait his turn and then distract him. You could ask Billy if he could let your child have a little turn for a while now or ask his parent to intervene. Once your toddler does get his turn with the toy, praise him again by saying something like, 'You were such a good boy for waiting so nicely. Now Billy has finished playing with the toy, it is your turn.'

Positive, calm reinforcement will always work much better in keeping your toddler calm and teach him that patience pays off. Sharing is an important skill to teach him, particularly in preparation for starting pre-school or nursery.

Dealing with fears

As your baby transitions to a toddler, he is learning so much about the environment around him. There is so much to take on board and it is very normal for him to be fearful of certain things or situations. The most common fears that develop in toddlers are:

- Fear of the dark and 'monsters' (see pages 29–36)
- Fear of loud noises he doesn't recognise
- Hand dryers in public toilets
- Bath/hair washing
- Insects (this may stem from a parental fear)
- Scary masks at Halloween or during dressing-up time
- Father Christmas or any dressed-up animals or characters you may see on an outing

Your toddler will grow out of most or all of the fears he develops, especially if he feels reassured by you when he becomes upset. If he shows fear of something, acknowledge it and calm him down. Say something like, 'It's okay, don't worry, it's not going to hurt you – Mummy is here to keep you safe.' Reassure him by showing that you aren't scared and your confidence over time will rub off on to him. If he's upset and scared and you show fear or, worse still, don't actually recognise and acknowledge his fear, then it won't help him in the long run. Telling him he shouldn't be scared or he should stop being so silly, doesn't give him the reassurance he needs.

As examples here are three fears that we have had to deal with regarding our toddler:

- *At around two years old our daughter developed a fear of having her hair washed and became scared about shampoo going into her eyes. I think it probably stemmed from Daddy bathing her one night and a little shampoo going into her eyes. After that night she decided that she didn't want to go back in the bath again as that would mean washing her hair. For a few nights just to get her to go in the bath, myself or my husband had to get in the bath with her. We agreed not to wash her hair at all and just made bathtime fun with toys and bath puzzles. This kept her relaxed and made bathtime enjoyable for her again.*

  A week in and her hair was looking like it needed a wash so again I got in the bath with her and mentioned that tonight we had to wash her hair. Immediately she began panicking and getting upset. I had a dry flannel ready and told her to put it over her eyes and lie back on me, and promised her that I would not get it into her eyes. I stayed calm, reassured her and just kept repeating, 'Mummy won't get it into your eyes.' Once I poured the first bowl of water over to wash the shampoo off and it didn't go in her eyes, I then had something to reassure her with: 'See, Mummy hasn't let it go in your eyes. Now lie still, good girl, nearly there,' and I continued reassuring and praising her. Once I'd finished, she sat up and praised me: 'Clever Mummy – not in my eyes.'

  Each time thereafter was a little easier as, although she would initially panic, I would just say, 'Mummy doesn't get it in your eyes – I didn't last time, did I?' Over one year later, she still gently reminds me before I begin to wash the shampoo off: 'Don't get it in my eyes, Mum,' and I always have to promise that I won't!

- *Hand dryers in public toilets can be very loud and to a toddler who is not used to standing in a confined space they can look, feel and sound truly terrifying. Our daughter became genuinely terrified of them when she came into the toilets with me. We began toilet training just after she turned two years old and if we were out and about and we went into a public toilet, she always refused to go near the hand dryer after she had washed her hands and used to tell me in a very sad voice that she didn't like it!*

  I would just say, 'Okay, you shake your hands dry and Mummy will use it to dry her hands.' I would then dry my hands under it with a big smile on my face and say things like, 'Oh it's nice and warm on my hands. It's not hurting Mummy is it? It's just drying my hands.' This is something I repeated each time we used a public toilet, to reassure her and I would always ask if she wanted to dry her hands under it too. One day she agreed to try and nervously put her hands close to it. I asked her if it felt cold or warm to distract her away from the fear and reassured her with praise for using the very noisy hand dryer. Like the hair washing, each time she used one it became easier and she was less fearful. Now aged almost four she loves hand dryers and has a massive smile on her face, laughing as she dries her hands, and even allows the warm air to blow on her face too!

- *My daughter was fearful of scary masks, as are many other toddlers. It is another very normal worry for toddlers, and is something especially likely to develop around Halloween. Most Halloween masks can be pretty gruesome, and if you have older children who think it is funny to wind their toddler sibling up by jumping out at them, then you have your work cut out not to be left with a screaming, terrified child by the end of the holiday period. Again, reassurance is the key and staying calm while showing your toddler that it is a mask. Encourage any siblings who may have scared him to lift the mask and show him their face saying, 'Look, it's Jack with a scary mask on.' Offer your toddler the opportunity to touch the mask while nobody is wearing it. Put it briefly on you and then lift it up quickly and say, 'Don't worry, it's just Mummy!' Your toddler may not want to touch it to begin with but eventually he will understand that it is only a mask and want to be involved in the game-playing side of it, although he may still become scared if he is not the one wearing it.*

Now my daughter is three years old, she will happily pick up and wear a Halloween mask and come up to me making 'roar' noises to try to scare me. I join in the game by saying, 'Argh scary, scary,' and cover my eyes. She will immediately take the mask off and say, 'Don't be scared, Mummy, it's just Loren,' and I will say, 'Oh okay, that's good then.'

Building confidence

How you react to the situations that arise over the next couple of years, as your toddler experiences new things, will make the vital difference to how confident or insecure he becomes as he gets older. Part of his experiences as a baby may have already paved the way, but his toddler years will be a vital time to encourage and build his confidence, so that he can learn to be more independent.

My top tips are:

- **Encourage independence:** Show him how to do things rather than doing them for him. This will help him learn to complete tasks independently and move on to the next stage of development. Practice makes perfect. If he is a particularly independent child anyway and won't let you show or help him, then back off a little. Let him try to do things alone and if you can see that he's struggling, say, 'That's a really good try. Shall I show you first or help you? Then you can do it without my help.' Wait until he's ready to accept your help – he has to learn to recognise when he does need help and over time will ask for it when he's struggling. If the task is really difficult, allow him to do the last bit of it, even if you are helping, so that he feels useful and involved. Then praise him: 'Wow, you did such a great job – thank you for helping me!'

- **Try not to show your fears:** To encourage confidence, independence and bravery in your toddler, you need to show enthusiasm and not be too over-protective. If there are certain things you are scared of, like heights or spiders for example, try not to show that in front of your toddler, or the same fears will pass over. *My mum is terrified of spiders and runs away when she sees the tiniest one – she always did this as I was growing up. I also have the same fear, although not quite as bad as her, as I'm happy to ignore tiny spiders, whereas she can't. Despite my fear and seeing spiders around the house on various occasions when my children have been home, I have always stayed calm and managed to either get Daddy to move the spider or removed myself and my toddler from the situation calmly, while reassuring them. None of my three children now have a fear of spiders. In fact my middle son quite happily goes and picks up the spiders in our house and puts them outside for me if Daddy isn't around to do it!*

- **Use siblings and other children's actions to your advantage.** For example, say, 'Wow, can you see what Jack is doing? Can you try that?' Toddlers love mimicking or copying other children.

- **Try not to use the word 'no' too often.** Instead explain why your toddler can't do something and then divert his attention to something else, thus avoiding a battle. 'Don't stand on the sofa – you might break it or fall off,' then lift him down and engage him in another activity straight away. Shouting at him to get down or telling him off may just result in a stand-off, which he will think is a great way to get lots of attention from you. He is more likely to do it again if he knows it winds you up! Keep things simple: give an instruction, then a reason for it, and encourage him to follow through and distract him straight afterwards to prevent a showdown.

- **Stay calm and positive:** If your toddler hurts himself, acknowledge it and cuddle and reassure him, but also keep a positive tone to your voice. If you are worried, then he will panic and become worried too. Even if there is blood and you are genuinely worried, it is important to reassure him to keep him calm. A magic kiss or rub usually works wonders with most toddlers!

Mummy's little helper

Toddlers love to help and be involved and busy a lot of the time. This may mean that your household jobs take a little longer than usual, as you have a very enthusiastic little person determined to help you with everything. Use it to your advantage and give your toddler little tasks to do. If he's busy and getting your attention, he will be happy. He's learning all the time and basic household jobs can aid his development in lots of ways – as well as increasing his confidence and independence, they can teach him about colours, shapes and amounts, and also develop his physical skills.

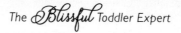

If he's scared, again reassure him and have cuddles but stay positive – try to make a joke out of the fearsome thing: For example, if he's scared of a hand dryer, say, 'Ooo look, it's blowing Mummy's hair.' Or if he's scared of a bug, say something like, 'Ooo look at its legs – how many has it got? More than you hasn't it!'

The bottom line is that if you are confident and show your toddler that it is okay and even exciting to try new things, he will develop into a confident person himself. Children learn by example.

Breaking bad habits

There are many different habits your toddler may develop that you find annoying and want to stop. In order to phase out a particular type of behaviour or habit, you first need to understand why or what may have triggered it to start. Various scenarios or feelings may prompt your toddler to engage in a bad habit as a form of comfort. Triggers include stress, insecurity, nervous feelings, being unhappy, bored, tired or as a means to fall asleep. Most of the time toddlers will grow out of the unwanted habit as they get older. Drawing too much attention to it by chastising, yelling or constantly requesting they stop may actually make the problem worse. Patience, praise, distraction and positive rewards and reinforcement will always work more effectively in your favour.

There are various types of behaviour that we have to teach our toddlers that are unacceptable – biting, hitting, pulling their trousers or skirt down in public, putting their hands down their trousers or knickers and also nose-picking.

Thumb-/finger-sucking

As a mother of two thumb-sucking children, I can tell you first hand that it has its pros and cons. The plus side is that it calms them in any situation, as it is a constant reassurance and comforter, even when a parent isn't around. The downside is that it is not something that can be taken away or stopped completely until your child is ready. Even then it may still be used into adulthood in relaxed situations – I even witnessed one of the dads I worked for suck his thumb while watching TV (I won't embarrass him by naming him publicly!)

With my eldest son we actually had an agreement between ourselves and our dentist that when he lost his top two baby teeth he would do his best to stop sucking his thumb. We talked about it for a good year before it happened to prepare him mentally and his top two teeth fell out within days of each other just before Christmas one year. We bought a product called 'Marvala stop', which is sold and promoted as something to paint on your child's thumb or fingers like a clear nail varnish, to stop thumb- or finger-sucking and nail-biting. It tastes dreadful and the idea is that as your child attempts to suck/chew his fingers, the taste will put him off until he no longer even attempts it.

Jack was in agreement that we should paint the solution on morning and night to help him stop sucking his thumb, and he willingly held it out for me to do it. The first week of bedtime settling was tough and we had a few tears as he found it much harder to settle to sleep without relying on his thumb, which he had used every night to settle for the last eight years. He felt determined, though, and with our praise and encouragement, after a few weeks, he told us that he was no longer even waking up sucking it early morning, which he had been doing when we first started applying the nail polish.

We thought we had cracked it. We had two whole months of no thumb-sucking day and night. And then Jack's baby sister was born, my third child. Roughly 2–3 weeks after her birth, I noticed that Jack had begun sucking his thumb again. I knew it was due to the new big change in our family and his insecurity and I didn't want to draw attention to it by going back to using the Marvala again while he was feeling insecure. Once things had settled down, I broached the subject with him again but he hasn't wanted to stop, so to be honest, I haven't pushed it. He is now 12 and still sucks his thumb at night and while relaxing in front of the TV, in the car, wherever he is when his hands aren't otherwise occupied, basically! However, he has naturally decided himself that it is not something he wants his friends to see him doing and hasn't sucked it at school for years, which tells me he is able to stop himself and control it when he wants to. I do tend to ask him to stop if he tries to talk to me with it in his mouth, or I feel he is doing it a little too much at times, but mostly I have just left him to it and hope one day he will grow out of needing to do it.

Dummies

If your toddler has had, and relied on, a dummy for sleep since being a baby, eventually there will come a point when you need to stop using it. Dummies generally cause unsettled sleep as your toddler will wake frequently to use the dummy to resettle himself. After doing this a number of times overnight, using the dummy as a sleep prop may not be enough any more and he may want you to help him get back to sleep. The faster you can phase out and stop dummy use the better – from a dental as well as sleep point of view. The longer your toddler uses a dummy, the more chance there is that the structure of the way the teeth come through the gums will be affected. This will, in turn, affect how his permanent teeth meet when he closes his mouth or bites as an older child or teenager.

The first thing I would suggest is to stop allowing him to have or hold it during the day for playtime and limit use only to naps and bedtime. Use a reward chart as an incentive for him to hand it to you in the mornings when he wakes up and at the end of any daytime naps. Once you reach the stage where you decide that it's time to stop using dummies altogether, the 'dummy fairy' is always the most effective method to use. How to implement this is described in detail on page 14.

Nail-biting

This is usually a habit connected to being nervous or bored. Distraction and reassurance as well as trying to keep your toddler busy will work best to break this habit, rather than telling him off. You can also try the Marvala nail varnish (see thumb-sucking, above), if the problem is really bad and he's making his finger sore and bleeding by biting the nail too low.

Nose-picking

Toddlers usually pick their nose because they have something up there bothering them. If they do it at home, it is less embarrassing to deal with. I usually say to toddlers, 'Take your finger out of your nose, please, and go and get yourself a tissue.' I ask if they have something up there and if they need help from me to get it, and then encourage them to wash their hands afterwards.

If you are out in public when the nose-picking starts, you will need to discourage the behaviour as a socially unacceptable thing to do. In public, I say to my toddler, 'Take your finger out of your nose, please – it's rude. If you need a tissue we can go to the toilet and find you one.' By offering a tissue as an alternative, you are acknowledging he may have a problem with something annoying up his nose, but also teaching him that he can't be dealing with it in that manner in the middle of a restaurant for example, while other people are eating. Have a conversation with him in the toilets: 'You mustn't put your finger up your nose while everyone is eating lunch – it's not very nice to watch. If you need a tissue, then you need to ask Mummy, please, and I will bring you to the toilet. Okay?'

Compare your toddler's behaviour to yours and to any siblings: 'You don't see Mummy picking her nose do you? Or Jack, or Ollie? No? You have to be a big boy like us and use a tissue, okay?' You then, of course, need to make sure you discourage any older siblings from nose-picking, as your toddler learns by example and will want to copy his siblings. If you are fairly firm in the no nose-picking while out socially, but allow your toddler to deal with any nose issues if he needs to in a private environment, then he will soon get the idea of when it is acceptable and when it is not.

Self-exploration

It is very normal for toddlers to put their hands down their trousers and touch themselves. This habit tends to be more common in boys. It can coincide with the beginning of toilet training as your toddler may enjoy running around with a minimal amount of clothing on, or even no clothes at all. Your job as a parent is to teach them that there are certain actions and behaviours that are not socially acceptable and cannot be done in the presence of others. Your toddler has to learn that there is a time and place for everything and maybe putting your hands down your pants in the lounge while Granny is visiting, isn't the right time.

On the occasions I have caught my boys doing it as toddlers, I have simply said, 'Take your hands out of your trousers, please. You mustn't do that when we have people here or we are out where other people can see you.' I then compare myself, husband and siblings and say, 'Mummy and Daddy don't do that when we are out do we? You don't see Jack putting his hands down his trousers when we have friends here to play do you?' It is something they can be directed to do while in the bath or in bed at night, for example. If you notice your toddler doing it at home when there is no one else there, then rather than telling them off, use your distraction skills to engage them in an activity. Self-exploration is usually linked to boredom, so if toddlers are kept busy they will be less likely to engage in it. Most children grow out of the habit very quickly if you don't make a big fuss about it.

Don't make your toddler feel that self-exploration is wrong altogether. It is perfectly natural for toddlers to explore themselves and important for them to understand their body and the differences there are between girls and boys. Answer any questions they ask with as much honesty as you can, without complicating things.

In our family my toddler realised very quickly that she was different to her brothers – bathtimes were hilarious when she was a baby and young toddler as she used to try and grab at her brothers, when she noticed they had something different to her. She was intrigued by it! She has understood from a young age that she and Mummy are girls and have a bottom and no willy, and Daddy and her brothers all have a willy and are boys. She knows that boys stand up when they have a wee but girls have to sit

down. I even 'test' her to see if she has understood the difference
by asking her about other family members and even pets, as to
whether she thinks they are boys or girls.

Biting

None of us want to be the parent whose toddler has just bitten
another child and made them cry. If you find your toddler is
regularly engaging in the cannibalism of their peers, then you
need to look at the possible causes of the behaviour before you
can stop it happening. It is actually a very common type of
behaviour in toddlers and below I have listed some of the reasons
it can happen – either as a one-off or as a regular occurrence:

- **Teething** – The molars and canines coming through cause
  pain and disruption between the ages of 1–3 years. This
  may make your toddler more likely to feel the need to chew
  on something. Offer him a cold flannel or even some of his
  favourite teething toys from when he was a baby to chew
  on and regular crunchy snacks, such as carrot, celery or
  cucumber with humous. Research has shown that soothing
  teething in this way can reduce biting incidents.
- **Lack of language skills** – if your toddler is frustrated
  and cannot vocalise his feelings, then biting can become
  a substitute for expressing anger and excitement, or even a
  way of letting people know they are too close.
- **Being overtired** – ensure your toddler is well rested before
  a social activity and encourage quality sleep overnight (see
  Chapter 1, Sleep Solutions).
- **Boredom** – use distraction and stimulate your toddler with
  engaging activities that keep him busy.
- **Experimenting** – he is biting to see how you will react.

Never bite back – yes, it would show your toddler how much biting hurts, but you can teach him that by allowing him to witness the reaction and upset his biting causes others. By biting him back you are reinforcing the behaviour rather than stopping it. How can you tell him not to bite if you do it to him when you are angry and don't like his behaviour or something he has done? That's exactly the reason he probably did it to one of his peers – because he didn't like what was happening during a social activity with his friends.

Instead keep your admonishment simple – no shouting or yelling. You can be firm and let your toddler know he is in the wrong without the need to shout. I know it's embarrassing but it's important you stay calm. Aggressive responses and harsh punishments to biting don't usually work – they will just increase your child's fear and anxiety, making him more likely to bite. A good response is to go up to your toddler immediately after and say in a firm voice, 'No biting. Biting hurts. Look at Ollie – he's crying because you hurt him and made him sad.'

You should then give the bitten child your attention (while keeping your toddler close to you by holding his hand to prevent him wandering off and attempting to do it again). Ask the bitten child if he's okay and make a fuss of him. This teaches your toddler that he won't get any attention for his behaviour. If your child is old enough and able to, encourage him to apologise. If not, do it for him. Once the bitten child has recovered, it's time to divert to a new activity, but before you begin you should remind your toddler that you don't want to see him biting any more as it's very unkind and makes everyone sad.

If you are the person who has been bitten, your initial reaction is likely to be a loud 'Ouch' or 'No' because it hurts! Your toddler will understand you are shocked and upset.

Once you have recovered, follow the guidelines above. Don't shout but be firm, then show your toddler that you are very sad and encourage him to give you a nice cuddle to make you happy again.

If you find that your toddler is becoming a regular biter, you need to look more closely at what triggers the biting:

- What was he doing at the time?
- What happened right before the biting incident?
- Is it always the same child he bites?
- Who was looking after your toddler? Was he at home or in a childcare setting?

Once you recognise the triggers, you can try to prevent the biting:

- **Keep a close eye on your toddler during play.** Be ready to step in if you see him becoming frustrated when a biting incident is more likely to happen.
- **Let him know you understand his frustration**, so he doesn't need to use biting as a way to explain his feelings: 'I know you want to have a turn in the car but Sophie is using it at the moment. It will be your turn soon.' Make sure he does then get a turn. Maybe use some sort of timer, such as an egg timer or the hands on a clock, that he can visually watch and wait for. Praise your toddler for waiting his turn or sharing and being kind to others: 'You are such a clever boy – you waited very nicely until it was your turn without pushing or biting. Good boy. High five me!'
- **If your toddler attends nursery or another childcare setting,** discuss any regular biting with them and ensure

that you are all handling it in the same way. Consistency and how you deal with it is the key to stopping any biting occurrences continuing.

While biting is very common, it usually stops by around three-and-a-half years old. If your toddler continues to bite regularly or the incidents are increasing rather than decreasing, despite you following the calm but firm response to any biting, it might be worth you asking your health visitor to refer you to a child development specialist for assessment, as there may be an underlying behavioural disorder that affects your child's normal social and emotional development.

Hitting

This is normal behaviour in toddlers linked to frustration at not being able to explain themselves clearly enough, or handle a difficult situation because they lack the maturity to do so.

As long as you are consistent and stay calm when your toddler hits you or another child, and teach him to be patient and gradually use his words when he is frustrated, he will stop hitting.

- Remember to be aware of potential triggers: tiredness and hunger can make a toddler less patient and more likely to lash out at you or others when he doesn't get what he wants.
- Teach him to 'use his words' to tell you or show you what he wants.
- Liaise with your toddler's other caregivers if he attends nursery or other childcare setting, so that you are all being consistent with boundaries.

Head-banging

This is fairly common – up to 20 per cent of babies and toddlers head-bang on purpose, with boys being more likely to do it than girls. It can start as young as six months and be at its peak between the ages of 18–24 months. The reasons for it tend to be:

- **Comfort:** Some toddlers find head-banging strangely comforting when they are tired or relaxed as they watch the TV. They may also bang their head in a rhythm to help themselves fall asleep at night-time.
- **Frustration:** Until your toddler has enough language development to express his needs and wants effectively, he can get very frustrated at not being understood. The head-banging may be part of a temper tantrum when he cannot get his own way.
- **Pain relief:** Some toddlers head-bang if they have teething or ear pain, as the motion can distract them from the pain.
- **To get attention:** If your toddler is bored and under-stimulated he may head-bang for attention. Because head-banging is something a parent wouldn't necessarily be comfortable seeing their child do, you will naturally give him the attention he craves, which encourages the behaviour even more.
- **A developmental problem:** Head-banging can be associated with developmental disorders such as autism if coupled with other signs and symptoms too. Head-banging alone does not indicate a developmental problem.

Try not not to draw attention to the head-banging as this will make your toddler more insecure and likely to increase how often he does it. Try to work out the triggers for the head-banging from the list above and act accordingly. Provide stimulating activities and give lots of attention when your toddler is not head-banging. If you notice that he does start doing it at any point during the day, distract him or encourage him to get involved in an activity with you, without actually making any reference to the head-banging you saw him doing.

Most will grow out of it fairly quickly within a few months, although for some it can go on longer. Chat to your health visitor or GP if you are worried that the head-banging is possibly linked to a developmental problem.

Imaginary friends

Don't worry if your toddler has an imaginary friend or animal that he seems to chat to and about all the time. Please feel reassured that it is a very normal part of development, with it being more common for a toddler to have one than not to.

Your toddler may name his friend and seem to be with them all the time, while others just crop up every now and then depending on your child's mood. Talking and interacting with an imaginary friend encourages language development, imagination and the skill to play independently without constant interaction from an adult. It doesn't make your toddler less likely to have friends and can in fact give him more confidence when in new situations with the silent knowledge that his imaginary friend is with him.

You may be wondering why your toddler has an imaginary friend when they have plenty of opportunity to socialise with others. There are a few possible reasons:

- Sometimes the firstborn in a family is more likely to have an imaginary friend or a younger child whose siblings are

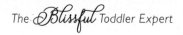

already attending school. It's an extra friend to play with whenever needed and one that your toddler has complete control over, who won't argue or disagree with the play choices he suggests.

- Imaginary friends can be a good way to comfort and reassure your toddler about his own fears. You may hear him saying, 'Don't worry, that noise won't hurt you,' and thus reassuring himself at the same time.

- Blaming an imaginary friend can be a good way to pass the blame for something that your toddler has done. You may ask 'Who made this mess?' and your toddler will reply something like, 'Not me – boy did it.'

Two out of three of my children have used imaginary friends as toddlers and pre-schoolers. My eldest had an imaginary friend called 'Boy' from when he was two until he started primary school. He would play with boy all the time at home and chat to him and tell me stories about the things he and boy did or would go and do. I used to encourage his talk to develop his vocabulary and imagination and, now he's at secondary school, people still comment on how much he talks and what a vivid imagination he has when he writes. My youngest uses her dolls as imaginary friends and carries two in particular around the house. She chats to them as she does various activities. I love to watch her involve them and also tell them off or reassure them about things when she feels necessary.

In short, don't worry. Relax and let your toddler enjoy playing with his special friend and use it as a learning experience to encourage his language and imagination. Most have usually stopped talking about their imaginary friend by the time they have finished their first year of primary school.

Feeling shy and encouraging friendships

If you have a particularly shy toddler, encourage his confidence and independence by allowing him to experience plenty of situations where he mixes with his peers – parks, toddler groups, singing and signing classes, for example. Interact with him and other children to support him at first, to show him how to approach others. Sometimes just making that first introduction can give your toddler the confidence to continue playing with other children and the more that grows, the better he will get at joining in and engaging with his peers more often without being shy.

Deciding what's acceptable

We all have various rules and expectations as parents and what you deem acceptable may not be what your best friend or sister will allow her children to do. Most of the boundaries and rules we encourage and teach our own children are based on how we ourselves were brought up. You may decide to instil the same ethics and standards of behaviour in your own children as you were taught, or decide to have either a more relaxed approach or stricter idea of parenting.

There is no right or wrong way to parent – as long as the basis of any decisions you make are in the best interests of your child and their welfare, safety and happiness, then that is what is important.

Table manners and what each parent expects from their children varies greatly – saying grace, eating with your mouth closed, holding your cutlery in a particular way and always sitting down together as a family to eat are just some things that different families feel are important table manners to instil in their children.

General manners include saying please and thank you, not interrupting adults while they are speaking, and excusing themselves if they 'burp' or 'trump'. The preferred word used for noises that come out of your bottom also varies greatly from family to family. Some parents are happy with the word 'fart', while others prefer words such as 'trumped' or 'popped'.

We all have different ages that we allow our toddler or older child to do things – having fizzy drinks and being allowed chewing gum are just two examples. You may see your neighbour's child regularly drinking coke or lemonade from the age of three but have decided you don't want your own children to do that until they are over the age of six – even then it will be a treat and not a regular everyday occurrence.

Changing the rules!

Your child's position in the family may also affect your parental decisions – many parents have far more relaxed rules by the time their second, third or even fourth child comes along, which can seem very unfair to your eldest, who remembers having to wait until he was much older before he was allowed to do certain things you now allow your toddler to do!

What you have to teach your child is that there may be different rules in certain situations or with particular caregivers. Grandparents, for example, are often more lenient. If my children stay at my parents' then I know for sure that they will get away with a lot more than they would at home – staying up late and eating more junk food and treats – but after all, isn't that what grandparents are for?

Most parents would agree that it is important to teach their toddler the basic manners of saying please and thank you, knowing (and using!) good table manners, and being respectful to adults, as part of developing good social skills in public for the future. If you instil those things from an early age by being a good example yourself, when your toddler is away from the family home and under the care or supervision of someone else, at nursery or with a childminder or relative, then he will remember those simple rules and boundaries you have taught him and make you proud.

However, it is perfectly normal for him to test the boundaries with you at home regularly. How will he learn just how far he can push you if he doesn't attempt various things? He has to learn at what point you tell him to stop doing things, in order to learn what is acceptable and what is not.

TIP

Consistency is the key. If you let him do something like climb on the table with his shoes on one day and then tell him off for it the following day, you will confuse him. He won't know if he's coming or going. To earn his respect, you need to decide on certain boundaries and consistently stick to them.

Is that my child?!

You may have friends and caregivers tell you how lovely your toddler is – for example, that he has good manners, is kind to other children, listens well – and you may actually wonder if they are really talking about *your* child!

At home he may at times be noisy, have tantrums and not listen to you, and you find you need the daily patience of a saint to keep up with him. You can't believe he could be so different away from home, right? Please be reassured that for 90 per cent of children and parents this is the case. They 'play up' for their parents and are like little angels away from them.

Shall I tell you why? (It's a good thing, don't worry.) It means you are doing a fantastic job at teaching your child boundaries and respect, which he uses to behave well when away from home. He knows right from wrong. He understands how to behave in certain situations all because you have taught him that.

We all need somewhere we can let off steam and/or someone to take our frustrations out on – for me it is usually my husband! If I'm tired or have had a busy day with the children, when he comes home from work it tends to be him that has to deal with a grumpy wife. It is usually the person closest to you, who you allow to see your frustration and vulnerability, because you know (or hope) that despite it, they love you enough to forgive you later on when you have calmed down.

For our children, *we* are that outlet. They play up with us and test us with challenging behaviour because, ultimately, they know we love them no matter what.

I remember my second son going through an insecure stage when his baby sister was born. He had just turned five years old and would constantly come up to me and tell me he loved me and want me to say it back. This would happen 10 or 20 times per day. He would then ask, 'Do you still love me, even when I do something naughty, Mummy?' I would reassure him and say, 'Of course I do. I don't like your behaviour sometimes but I will always love you no matter what.' With constant reassurance, he grew out of it and stopped asking eventually.

This is what toddlers are testing – your patience and your love for them. When they are away from home, they don't have that same connection with their caregivers. Toddlers want to be liked, they want others, especially adults, to be happy with them and they very quickly learn that their behaviour needs to *be* likeable to make the adults around them happy.

If your toddler behaves well for everyone else apart from you, give yourself a huge pat on the back. You may not realise it, but he is taking everything that you teach him on board and using those boundaries in other social situations. It means you are doing a great job as a parent. I didn't fully understand this until I had children myself, and that is why I find it difficult to take advice, on behaviour in particular, from any parenting expert who doesn't actually have children themselves.

I worked as a nanny for years before I had children and was aware that the children in my care always behaved much better for me than they did their parents. With my non-parent judgemental head on, I used to think, when I have children I will make sure I bring them up not to talk or act in certain ways I witnessed my nanny children behaving towards their parents.

One particular incident sticks in my mind …

CASE STUDY: Alex

I used to look after a three-year-old boy called Alex and he was the most placid, compliant, agreeable toddler to look after. I never had to tell him off at all – he always did exactly as I asked whenever I wanted him to and was a joy to look after. One evening his mum came home from work and I was busy upstairs putting some washing away, but heard her come in. Alex had been happily playing downstairs and the next thing I heard was him shouting and crying, so I went running down the stairs and found him at his mother's feet having a full-blown tantrum. I was shocked – I had never seen him act this way or even raise his voice. I asked her what had happened and she said he had asked if he could go and watch some TV. She had said no, maybe after his bath, and the result was an angry toddler on the floor at her feet!

The mother could obviously see I was shocked at Alex rolling around on the floor and said, 'Doesn't he do this for you?' I replied, 'No, he never even says no to me – he doesn't give me any trouble at all,' to which she answered, 'Oh you wait until you have your own children!'

Two years later when I had my own toddler, I realised how right Alex's mum's warning was! For the most part my children are fairly well behaved – particularly my toddler as she hasn't started school yet and developed what I like to call 'the school yard attitude'. Her brothers aged eight and 12 do have the ability to push their luck on a regular basis with back chat and by making things difficult on occasions – for example, when we are all trying to rush out the door for school in the mornings.

However, I am very proud to say that they are kind, polite, caring children when they are at school and at friends' or relatives' houses. They show other adults the respect they have been taught and I always get such lovely feedback from any adult they have spent time with. This proves to me, no matter how much I doubt myself daily, that I am doing a good job, as my children know how to behave in various social settings and situations.

This is what I tell all parents that I work with or meet, who are worried about their child's behaviour. It is normal for children to test the boundaries and show their frustrations at home, but if their behaviour elsewhere is (for the most part) very good, then you are heading in the right direction with the lessons you teach them.

If, however, your toddler is misbehaving outside of the home – at nursery or pre-school when away from you – then you need to look at the triggers and reasons why that may be the case. It could be due to family circumstances changing, for example:

- Death in the family
- Marriage break-up
- New sibling
- Moving house
- Something more complicated, and linked to a developmental or behavioural problem, such as autism or ADHD, for example. If you are concerned that your toddler's behaviour doesn't seem to be improving, despite you setting consistent boundaries, and other childcarers are also finding your child's behaviour hard to manage, it's worth having a chat to your health visitor or GP about your concerns.

Tantrums in public

Like most parents, you may worry about how to handle a public tantrum. It's normal to feel embarrassed and that your parenting skills are being judged by onlookers. For the most part, a full-blown tantrum can be avoided if you follow these tips:

- **Ensure your toddler is well rested** before you attempt a shopping trip or activity you know is difficult at the best of times. A tired toddler will not be a very patient one and a busy shopping trip won't be much fun for a toddler who is not in the mood to be there.
- **Keep your toddler busy** and engaged with talk while you're out and about. If he's busy chatting and looking

around while talking to you about his environment, he's less likely to get bored and have a tantrum.

- **Involve him.** If you are shopping, give him his own list of items to find.
- **Offer an incentive** before you go out to a public place. Tell your toddler he will be rewarded for good behaviour at the end of the outing. Remind him of this during the outing and praise good behaviour while you are out to help spur him on to continue behaving well.

If, despite your best efforts, a tantrum seems to be starting due to your toddler wanting something he can't have or something not going quite his way, now is the time to get your best distraction skills going. Get down to his level, explain to him why he can't have or do something and then immediately distract him with something else you have seen or talk about an activity he did earlier that day or is going to be doing soon. Do not give in to tantrums. If you have said no to something then stick to it, otherwise your toddler will know how to get you to change your mind next time with a little bit of kicking and screaming. Remind him of your initial promise of a treat for good behaviour and that if he can't listen to you now and continue helping you and behave well, then he won't earn that treat that was originally promised.

If you are in a restaurant you can always take your toddler to the toilets or outside and have a private conversation with him away from the public eye. Usually the time out away from everyone is enough to calm the situation and remind your toddler that you won't tolerate bad behaviour and that he will miss out on the family activity if he chooses to continue behaving badly.

Swearing

A toddler's language can develop very quickly and, without you realising it, your toddler will suddenly be listening to everything you say, good and bad – and repeating it! Despite the fact my children may hear my husband or me swear on occasion, they have learnt that we are adults and therefore *allowed* to swear if we want to. I believe it is important that children learn there are different ages and stages that they get to do things, such as walking without holding your hand on an outing, going to the toilet alone, crossing the road alone, drinking fizzy drinks, etc.

Swearing is one of those activities, like driving, smoking and drinking alcohol, that children have to realise that only adults can do. They may see or witness us do all of those things but that doesn't mean that they are old enough, or allowed, to do them.

My eldest two boys hear swearing from the adults around them but they know that it is something I don't ever expect to hear from them. I understand that one day, when they are out with their mates, they will think it makes them look big and clever to use the odd swear word. However, I have taught them that they should never use swear words in the presence of another adult or a child much younger than them.

Unfortunately, your toddler will not understand all of this yet. He hears words and will repeat them. He will not understand what they mean and that some words are good and some are not so nice to repeat at the top of his voice in the middle of the supermarket! It is for this reason I would recommend that you try to stop yourself from swearing in your toddler's presence, to prevent an embarrassing occasion. Until my children understood the whole concept of swearing, which was around the age of five years old, my husband and I have tried not to swear in front of them.

My husband learnt this the hard way when our firstborn picked up the 'f word' from him during a stressful football game he had been watching on the TV. The next time Jack was sat on the silly step for something, he began shouting it at the top of his voice. He used it in exactly the right context. The amazing thing was that he never said it to our face, only to vent frustration when he couldn't see us. We decided not to make any reference to it, or mention it when we took him off the stairs at the end of his time out. It was at that moment that my husband realised that he had to completely stop swearing in front of him. The swearing on the stairs then stopped after a couple of weeks.

Now with our third child going through her toddler language stages, we are very aware that we don't want to swear in front of her, so we both tend to use other words in place of swearing. 'Fudge', 'sugar' and 'for goodness' sake' to name a few – all of which I have heard my daughter use, in the right context, when she gets annoyed with something. Therefore I am grateful that she isn't hearing anything worse.

If you do happen to swear and your child copies, the best thing you can do is *not* react to it. Don't tell him off, don't draw attention to the word as that is a surefire way to get him repeating it over and over again for attention. If he is repeating the swear word, try to distract him with something else in the hope that he will forget the lovely new word he has just learnt!

An older toddler (around four years old) who is bright, is likely to know you are trying to fool him, so that will be the time to explain that there are some words grown-ups say that children shouldn't. Apologise for saying it and explain that Mummy was a bit silly for saying it and you will try not to say it again. Tell him that if you do swear he is allowed to tell you off or even send you to the silly step. It will make him feel important and also create a little more respect between you both, as you admit that you are sometimes wrong too.

Twins

Twins, just like all siblings, will develop and learn things at a different rate. Even if you have identical twins I am sure that you have already noticed by the time they reach toddlerhood, they are very individual and have developed and achieved milestones at separate times and are likely to even have very different personalities.

You may have one twin who is the more dominant, confident one who is 'allowed' by their sibling to lead the way. Equally, both may have very dominant personalities that makes sharing a difficult and stressful daily occurrence for everyone. If you are busy doing something with one twin, the other one may start to misbehave to get your attention. If you are distracted with household chores while they are seemingly happy playing together nicely, they may both start to misbehave to get your attention. Trying to give both children equal attention is one of the biggest challenges for parents of twins.

The best piece of advice I can give you with twins is, if finances allow, buy two of everything, once they reach the toddler years. Why should they be forced to share toys from a very young age just because they were born at the same time as another person? Buy two dolls, two trains, two diggers, two colouring sets. If they have one each, then it will go some way to stopping the constant fighting.

Once they know they have the same things, there will be less fighting. If, however, your twin still wants the toy his

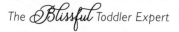

brother or sister is playing with, use your distraction skills. Offer alternatives and use the praise and reward techniques explained earlier in this chapter or time out if necessary.

With twins I always find you can use the good behaviour of one to encourage the other to stop being silly: 'Wow, look how nicely Jack is playing. Shall we go and see if we can find a toy and join in?' If your toddler doesn't want to do as you suggest initially, leave him to contemplate: 'Okay you stay there. I'm going to go and play with Jack and you can come over when you want to join in and have fun with us.' Use an enthusiastic voice during play with the other twin to draw the grumpy one back over to play. You should find that very quickly he won't be able to resist joining in, as he won't like feeling he is missing out on any attention. If you find they have occasions where they are both misbehaving and you need to use time out, it's advisable to establish and have separate areas for them in different rooms, so that they both have time to calm down during their time out period, without the distraction of their sibling.

Special needs children

Many children with special needs have behavioural issues that are part of their diagnosis. They may not do what you want or need them to due to impulses or self-protective routines that we may find hard to understand. That doesn't mean you have to accept aggression, chaos and rule-breaking as part of everyday life, but you do have to work harder to find a balance and compromise that works.

The first thing you need to do is to understand your child's special needs, any diagnosis and what that could mean both in the short and long term. Once you do, moving forward in a slow and consistent way is the next step.

How you react to certain situations will make the vital difference to how your toddler responds. Patience, perseverance and consistency are even more essential in dealing with behavioural issues with many special needs children, as any change to a routine can affect behaviour dramatically.

If you do suspect that your child has a behavioural or developmental delay or disorder, you should firstly speak to your GP or health visitor for a diagnosis. If a condition is diagnosed, there are lots of amazing support groups, charities and organisations, where you will find more information to help your child develop to his full potential. These have been listed at the end of the book on pages 307–9.

It's important to liaise with all of your toddler's caregivers so that you are all consistently giving the same message to combat any difficult behaviour.

Introducing a new sibling

No matter how much you try to prepare your toddler for the arrival of a new baby brother or sister, he is still going to get a pretty big shock when your new little bundle of joy arrives. His whole world as he knows it is going to completely change. He will no longer have the undivided attention of two parents. Suddenly there is a new person he has to share you with. To make matters worse, to begin with this new person isn't that much fun – all he does is cry, feed, poo and sleep!

Preparing your toddler for the new arrival while you are pregnant is essential. *Having had three children myself, I have had to prepare older siblings twice for a new arrival and I'm proud to say my toddlers' reaction to the new baby has never been anything but love and affection towards their new sibling. We had a few behavioural issues (discussed on pages 74–80) directed at myself and my husband and the boundaries were well and truly tested once the baby arrived, but no aggression or animosity was ever shown towards the baby. I'm certain that was due to the preparation we put in before the baby arrived and all the praise and attention given afterwards.*

Preparation

To prepare your toddler for the arrival of his new baby sibling:

- **Discuss the impending arrival,** but not too early on in the pregnancy – toddlers have no sense of time and nine months is a long countdown. Wait until you start to get a bigger pregnancy tummy before talking about the new baby.
- **Use event milestones** to discuss when the baby will arrive – for example, after Christmas time or after Mummy and Daddy have both had our birthdays, then it will be time for the baby to come.
- **Encourage your toddler to talk to the baby** in your tummy and feel it kick. Give praise and reassurance when he does and tell him how much the baby loves hearing his big brother talk. It's also important not to force him, though. If he doesn't want to, then that's okay.
- **Suggest he helps you get things ready for the baby,** such as choosing special outfits or cuddly toys from the shop, or even helping Daddy put the new cot up or other baby equipment. These can be used positively when the baby arrives: 'Wow, she's wearing the top you chose for her – I think she loves it. You made a good choice.'
- **Talk about what will happen when the baby arrives,** where the baby will sleep, how you will feed – whether

breast- or bottle-feeding – and how you would love it if your toddler would help you look after the baby.

- **Buy a doll or teddy and teach your toddler how to role-play** and be gentle with it. Teach him how to burp it, feed it and he could even practise putting one of the newborn nappies you have for the baby on to the doll or teddy. He can then be encouraged to play and engage with the doll or teddy at the same time as you are feeding or changing the baby when it arrives, and also whenever you or Daddy are changing the baby's nappy.

- **Buy or borrow children's books about Mummies having babies** as the birth approaches. Reading these to your toddler will help him understand the whole concept.

- **As the birth gets closer, make sure he is aware what will happen.** If you choose to have a home birth, explain it in simple terms and if a hospital birth is likely, reassure him and let him know who will be caring for him when the time comes.

Once the baby arrives

- **It's a good idea to buy a special present** you can give to your toddler from the new baby. It can be presented to your toddler the first time he meets his new sibling, so either while you are still in hospital or on the day you bring the new baby home. Your toddler is likely to be very curious when he meets the new baby for the first time.

- **Remind your toddler that he needs to be gentle** like he is with his baby doll or teddy. If he wants to hold the baby, sit him down and let him – give him help and support and lots of praise for holding the baby so well. Remind him that he needs to support the baby's head carefully at all times.

You can use cushions to help him or support with your arm if needed. Reassure him that the baby loves having a cuddle with his big brother.

- **Remember that newborn babies are much more robust than they look**, so try not to pick up on your toddler being a little less delicate than you would like. If he is being a little rough and you feel you do need to say something, use positive praise: 'Wow, you are doing so well – just hold her head a little bit more for Mummy, that's it, good boy. She would like it if you stroked her face gently. I don't think she wants you to pat her or poke her – just nice stroking. Good boy.'

- **Try to make time for your toddler to hold the baby** whenever he asks. If you are feeding the baby, agree that he can hold her afterwards. Try not to discourage any loving attention he shows towards the baby, as he will stop asking if you do and negative thoughts are more likely to slip in.

- **Encourage him to help you care for the baby** – fetching things and helping to clean, feed or wind the baby. A toddler's concentration span for an activity doesn't always last that long so he will probably only want to help for a few minutes and will then resume playing.

- **Try to make time for your toddler every day** without the baby being present. If you are on your own all day with both baby and toddler, this can still be done by simply putting the baby down for a nap in another room – or at least in a Moses basket or cot away from you. It is important your toddler still has special one-to-one time with Mummy and Daddy individually without the baby present, to stop any resentment or animosity developing. Let him see both of you spend time with the baby and equally share your time with him too, so that he doesn't feel left out.

- **When you are feeding the baby,** try to sit and play with your toddler and engage him in an activity that will keep him busy. However, if he would rather sit with you, have a selection of special books that you can bring out, so that your toddler doesn't feel left out as you feed.

- **When visitors come,** try to ensure they give your toddler attention first and don't just head straight for the baby. Encourage them to ask your toddler to show them the baby. If they bring a present for the baby they can also be encouraged to bring something for the new big brother too, even if it is something small like a favourite magazine or treat. This is easier to ask of close friends and family, of course. Most visitors will naturally involve your toddler and chat to him about being an older sibling. If they don't, try to give your toddler lots of attention so that he doesn't end up feeling left out by all the attention the baby is getting.

Behaviour

The biggest thing you are likely to notice a week or two after the baby arrives, when the novelty has worn off and your toddler has realised this new little person is here to stay, is that his behaviour may become more testing. He may do things that he knows are usually not allowed, say things he shouldn't and just generally try to push his luck and wind you up. The family dynamics have changed so all he is doing is checking if the rules have changed too.

Although it is important to understand and empathise that he has had a massive change in his life, it's important that you are still consistent with rules and boundaries. What he needs most is for everything else he is used to doing, to remain as normal as possible. That will reassure him that everything else will also settle down as you all get used to each other.

You may find in the days and weeks after the baby is born that your toddler shows a preference for one parent or the other and want that one to do everything for him. It may be Daddy because he has noticed how busy Mummy is with the baby, particularly if you are breastfeeding and doing the bulk of the baby care. However, it may be that your toddler suddenly wants you to do everything for him as a means to draw you away from the baby. Reassure him, make time for him as much as you can and he will soon settle down.

As your new baby begins to smile and develop a personality, you are likely to find that all of her best smiles and giggles are saved for her older sibling – at times without any interaction needed at all. She will follow him around the room with her eyes and enjoy watching him play. This is the time that toddlers can really be encouraged to interact with their new sibling and they will love the fact they can make the baby smile and laugh. You get to reap the rewards and enjoy watching the bond they build and that's what it's all about.

Of course there are going to be times that your toddler may not want the baby around, especially if it stops you participating in an activity with him. Problems may also start when his new sibling has learnt to crawl. A crawling baby brother or sister doesn't tend to have a lot of respect for a Lego castle or newly set-up train track or doll's house, which your toddler may have spent a long time perfecting.

It is important to give your toddler time to play with his toys alone or with you, without the baby destroying his toy set-up. If you play with him, you can stop any aggression developing from your toddler's frustrations at his newly mobile sibling.

By following all of these tips as closely as you can, the transition from one to two children, or introducing a new sibling to a toddler at any point in the family dynamics, should only ever be a positive, happy experience for all of you.

Regression

*When a new baby arrives, it is very normal for a toddler to regress a little in terms of development. He may say he wants to drink from a bottle like the baby, or for you to cuddle him like a baby cradled in your arms. Wanting to sit in the baby's chair or climb in the cot are also very common types of toddler behaviour at this stage. Your toddler is naturally just trying to get your attention. For some things you can role-play and indulge him, such as cradling him like a baby or pretending to wrap him up like the baby. The best way to deal with this behaviour is to remind your toddler of all the interesting things the baby **can't** do, such as eat and drink nice things, run around and play with toys, etc. This will encourage your toddler to continue wanting to act more maturely.*

It is also very normal for a little regression to occur with toilet training. As long as you stay relaxed and only ever positive then any regression will soon settle down as your toddler feels more secure. If you plan on a big transition, such as starting toilet training or moving your toddler from a cot to a bed, try to do this 3–6 months before the new baby arrives to ensure your toddler is happy and settled before the new baby is born.

What if you need a break?

I love having my toddler daughter help me with household chores most of the time. It keeps her busy, she gets so excited that she's allowed to help, and we have great conversations as each task turns into a whole learning experience. However, there are times where I need to get something done super-fast and I don't have the extra time it will take if she helps me. There are also times when I just need five or 10 minutes to myself to re-energise or calm down if we have had a particularly trying morning or afternoon and my patience has been tested repeatedly.

These are the times I enlist the help of the TV or tablet. In my opinion, as long as your toddler isn't constantly using them, it is perfectly okay to use them in moderation. Many apps and TV programmes are very educational these days so your toddler can actually be learning while you have your five- or 10-minute break.

My daughter has two particular favourite programmes and I know that if I put an episode of one of those on it will 'buy' me 10 whole minutes of quiet time. It's truly amazing how much you can get done in 10 minutes without a toddler in tow – the washing machine and dishwasher can be unloaded and even the washing hung out on the line. If I had a toddler helping then each of those tasks would have likely taken me 10 minutes, so if I'm in a rush, it is helpful to have the option of the television. Alternatively, the 10 minutes while your toddler is quiet can be used to take a break yourself and have some time out to re-energise in another room. It's amazing how a short rest period can give you the extra patience you need to make it through to bedtime on a challenging day with your toddler.

There are various apps that my toddler also loves to play – a memory card matching game and also a party time one that gives her verbal instructions she has to follow and click on certain things. Again, these are activities she doesn't need my presence for. We have done them so many times together that she can now manage them alone.

Of course while I'm running around like a headless chicken, as she sits in front of the TV or tablet, I check on her regularly – it's amazing what an unsupervised toddler can get up to in as little as five minutes. If you ever meet my husband, then ask him about our daughter and a bottle of suncream!

Sometimes, as parents, we need that five or 10 minutes to sit down. It doesn't make you a bad parent. In fact I think recognising that *you* need a time out actually makes you a better parent than you otherwise would be. It gives you time to find a little more energy for all those questions, a little more patience for the testing behaviour you encounter with a toddler and that ultimately can only benefit your child.

So, recognise and take time out when you need it. Find an activity that your child loves and get it set up to 'buy' you that time out. It may not be the TV or tablet. It may be that you can set up a doll's house that will occupy your toddler for 10 minutes or a train or car track. Whatever it is, use that time to grab those last reserves that you need to get you through the rest of the day until bedtime.

TIP

If it's a longer break you need, then consider asking friends or relatives for help – maybe start a babysitting circle, so that you can all have time off every now and then – during the day or evening. A haircut appointment or even shopping alone can make you feel better. If you return the favour, then others will be willing to help.

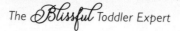

Parenting is the hardest job in the world – it's okay to ask for help and it's okay to plan the odd hour, morning or even evening off. Recognising that you need time out every now and then will only make you a better parent during the quality time you do spend with your children and being a good parent is all each of us can strive to be.

As a parent, you are the greatest influence on your toddler's behaviour and development. It is hard work but as always P&P – patience and perseverance – will be your most valuable tool. Remember to use these, plus be consistent when things are tough. And also remember, there is no way to be a perfect parent – but a million and more ways to be a good one!

4

Speech and language

Hearing your baby begin to develop speech is one of the most wonderful parts of parenthood. As your baby transitions to a toddler, it is her speech development that begins to shape the person she is – it will be a wonderful experience to watch her personality develop alongside her speech. As she learns new words and how to communicate her needs verbally, you will feel very proud. It is also the time to begin watching *what* you say too – toddlers learn very quickly, and not always words or phrases that you want them to (see page 115)! Hearing your toddler come out with some of the regular phrases you or your partner use can be a funny and sometimes eye-opening experience. Sometimes we don't actually realise how much we use a certain word or phrase until we hear our toddlers begin to use the same one in the correct context!

There are many things that can influence and determine how quickly your child's speech develops as she transitions from being a baby to a toddler:

- Home environment
- How many languages are spoken at home
- Position in the family

- Special needs
- Reliance on a dummy or sucking her thumb/fingers

These factors are all discussed within this chapter but the biggest influence, which trumps all others, is how much time you spend trying to encourage your toddler's speech development.

Encouraging speech development

Understanding always comes first. If you spend time every day talking to your toddler about anything and everything she will constantly be hearing speech and be encouraged to begin to communicate back to you in some way. She will gain confidence and her language skills will develop naturally over time. To encourage speech development:

- **Give her tasks to do** so that she learns to understand and follow instructions. For example, say, 'Go and put that in the bin, please. Can you go and get the ball?' If she understands and can follow simple instructions, that is half the battle.
- **Talk to your toddler as you are doing things** and give her the opportunity to respond: 'Mummy is putting the washing on. Can you say "washing"? Mummy is making you a drink. Can you say "drink"?' Even if her attempts at words are not clear or recognisable to begin with, the fact that she is trying to vocalise should be praised. That will encourage her to continue trying and with practice she will improve.
- **Read picture books and simple word books** together. Point out objects and encourage your toddler to repeat words after you, or ask her to point out the objects that you ask for. This is a fun activity that encourages learning and speech. You can also do this with objects around the house,

asking your toddler to fetch you things or repeat words you say. Always praise her when she tries.

- **Sing songs and basic nursery rhymes** – it is a brilliant way to encourage speech and the repetition helps to reinforce vocabulary and they show how rhythm and inflection is used in speech. Short, repetitive rhyming stories do the same too.

- **Play games and make talking and learning fun**. As your toddler's speech develops and improves, you can begin to teach her to count and learn the alphabet too, in preparation for starting nursery and school. Learning about various colours and the use of similar describing words such as 'big', 'huge' and 'massive' during activities will all help to increase her vocabulary on a daily basis.

Rate of speech development

Toddlers develop speech at a different rate. Some have a wide range of vocabulary by two years of age, while others will be barely saying a word. As long as your toddler understands and can follow simple instructions, the actual speech and language will come with time – you just need to continue to encourage it every day and give your toddler opportunities to vocalise.

All three of my children have been very different in their rate of speech development. My eldest was very advanced with speech and you could easily hold a conversation with him by the time he was two years old. In contrast, my second son was the opposite and much slower at everything in comparison to his brother – teething, crawling, walking and talking. To be honest because I had two children and my toddler was very loud, vocal and demanding, my younger son just happily fitted in and followed his brother around. I unfortunately had less time than I would have liked to spend encouraging his language and any time he did make any attempt to talk or vocalise his needs or wants, my eldest son would end up pointing out what he wanted and 'talking' for him. Once my eldest went off to school, I had much more time to devote to my second son and his speech came on and improved very quickly.

My youngest daughter was born after my second son had already started school so she has always had me to herself during the day, while her big brothers attend school. This individual attention has meant that, like her eldest brother who had the same, she has had an amazing language base from 18 months and it has been easy for anyone to understand what she says from the age of just over two.

Pronunciation

It's normal for toddlers to pronounce words incorrectly to begin with. Don't react negatively to this as it may discourage your toddler from even attempting to talk. You can encourage correct pronunciation by simply repeating words back to her in the correct way, without actually telling her she has pronounced them wrong. For example, if she says, 'Dink pease,' then you repeat, 'Drink please? Is that what you would like Mummy to get you?'

If your toddler has a dummy or sucks her thumb, this may affect the way she pronounces words, especially if she regularly tries to talk with her thumb or dummy in her mouth. Always discourage this and ask her to take her thumb/dummy out, as you can't hear what she is saying. Then ask her to repeat what she said. Initially, she may still say the word as if the dummy or thumb is still in her mouth. Just repeat it in the correct way and she will pick this up over time as her use of the dummy or thumb reduces.

All three of my children have had initial problems with pronunciation as two of them sucked their thumbs and one had a dummy. My elder two progressed to gradually pronouncing words correctly with encouragement by the time they started school, and my youngest is almost there too. I find with her it's more forgetfulness and that she says a word as if she has her thumb in her mouth. However, if I ask her to repeat it properly then she can make the sounds she needs to.

As children learn to talk, the speed at which they learn different sounds develops gradually, with some developing earlier than others. As a guide, the table below shows the ages that sounds develop by (where English is the first language spoken at home).

Approx age	Usually children will:
18–24 months	Use a limited number of sounds in their words, often these are 'p', 'b', 't', 'd', 'm' and 'w'. At this age children will often miss the ends off words. They can usually be understood about half of the time.
2–3 years	Use a wider range of speech sounds. However, many children will shorten longer words, such as saying 'nana' instead of 'banana'. They may also have difficulty where lots of sounds happen together in a word, e.g they may say 'pider' instead of 'spider'. They often have problems saying more difficult sounds like 'sh', 'ch', 'th' and 'r'. However, people that know them can mostly understand them.
3–4 years	Have difficulties with a small number of sounds – for example, 'r', 'w', 'l', 'f', 'th', 'sc', 'ch' and 'z'.
4–5 years	Use most sounds effectively. However, they may have some difficulties with more difficult words such as 'scribble' or 'elephant'.

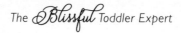

> ### TIP
>
> *If you are at all worried about your child's speech or hearing, have a chat with your GP or health visitor, who will refer you to a specialist, if necessary.*

Glue ear

Repeated middle ear infections may lead to glue ear, where sticky fluid builds up and can affect your child's hearing. This may lead to unclear speech and behaviour problems. It is estimated that 1 in 5 children around the age of two years old will be affected by glue ear at any given time and about 8 in every 10 children will have had glue ear at least once by the time they are 10 years old. More details on glue ear and the causes, symptoms and treatment are discussed on page 228.

CASE STUDY: Lucy

At age 2 Lucy was trying to talk but her speech wasn't very clear, so her mum, Rachael, consulted a health visitor. Up to that point Rachael had put Lucy's unclear speech down to dummy use, which was then stopped on her birthday using the dummy fairy (see page 14). The health visitor advised Rachael to see a GP, who referred Lucy for a hearing test. Glue ear was diagnosed. It had affected the way Lucy heard sounds and that was why she wasn't as clear in her own speech.

Lucy had grommets fitted just before her fourth birthday and was booked in for speech therapy sessions. She would have a six-week block of one-to-one speech therapy and then have a break for a month or two, then another six-week block. Rachael was doing one-to-one speech therapy at home, too, as advised by the therapist and once she started school they were also doing the same. Lucy was very shy outside of the family home and wouldn't interact with any other adults or answer them if they spoke to her, so one-to-one therapy was essential. Rachael had to keep reminding Lucy to use her big voice that she used at home.

At pre-school she would interact and talk to other children but not adults. She would do what they asked, follow direction and understand, but she just wouldn't answer if they ever spoke to her and wanted her to respond to a question they asked. After a few months of being at school in the reception class Lucy's confidence began to grow and by the age of six, when she had moved into year one, her speech was much clearer and the once shy little girl who wouldn't talk to any adults will now confidently reply.

Bilingual children

If you and your partner speak two different languages, try to stick to one language each so as not to confuse your toddler. She will very quickly learn that one form of communication and language is associated with Mummy and a different one with Daddy.

Sometimes parents are discouraged from using two languages at home. They're told it can lead to confusion and speech delays, or that they've missed the window of opportunity. Some parents think that if a child is exposed to two languages at the same time, she might become confused and not be able to differentiate between them. This is totally incorrect.

'From just days after birth, all infants can tell the difference between many languages,' says Barbara Zurer Pearson, author of *Raising a Bilingual Child*. She says this is especially true when the languages are quite different from each other – as different, for example, as French and Arabic. 'At that young age, infants generally still have trouble telling two very similar languages apart, like English from Dutch. But by about six months of age, they can do that too,' she says.

Children raised in a bilingual household with at least two languages being spoken at home tend to begin speaking a little later than their peers. The delay is only temporary though and, according to experts, not a general rule. If there is an initial delay, by the time they start school the children who speak more than one language are on par or even ahead of their peers in regard to language skill. It's never too late – or too early – to introduce your child to a second language.

Pearson says, 'Learning a second language is easier for children under 10, and even easier for children under five, compared with the much greater effort it takes adults.' The optimal time, according to experts, seems to be from birth to 3 years – exactly when a child is learning her first language, and her mind is still open and flexible. The next best time for learning a second language appears to be when children are between 4 –7 years old, because they can still process multiple languages together and continue to build a second language alongside the first and learn to speak both languages fluently.

If your child is older than seven, and you've been thinking about raising him bilingually, it's still not too late. The third best time for learning a second language is from about age eight to puberty. After puberty, studies show, new languages are stored in a separate area of the brain, so children have to translate or go through their native language as a path to the new language. 'We hear so much about the special "window of opportunity" for young children to learn two languages that it can be discouraging to the older child,' says Pearson. 'It's true that it's easier to start earlier, but people can learn a second language even after the window has closed.'

Twins

If you have twins you will have learnt by now that they develop at their own rate and being a twin, whether identical or fraternal, does not mean they will do or learn things at the same time. Speech and language is just another one of those things that they will develop individually. Many twin parents actually find that one twin is more vocal than the other, and that is very normal. You may also notice that they have their own 'language' that they use to communicate with each other. You may not understand it but they will know exactly what it means and you may have one twin who will 'speak for' their sibling regularly when they are first learning to talk. This scenario can also occur in siblings who are not twins, but very close in age.

Stammering

It's very normal for toddlers to have a slight stammer as they rush to tell you something and can't get the words out quickly enough. This can cause them to stammer or stutter their words and is known as 'developmental stammering'.

The following information is taken from the NHS Direct website: 'Stammering is common in young children. Estimates for developmental stammering vary, but it is expected that 5–8 per cent of pre-school age children will experience a phase of non-fluent speech. The condition is more likely to persist in males than females, which is why there are four times more men than women with a stammer. The reason for this is unclear. All ethnic groups are affected equally by stammering. The causes of stammering are still uncertain, but evidence suggests that inheriting certain genes may increase a child's likelihood of developing a stammer.'

Treating stammering

According to the NHS Direct website, around three in four cases of developmental stammering in pre-school children will resolve without treatment. One in four children will need therapy to stop a persistent stammer developing. Treatment is highly successful in resolving stammers in pre-school age children, especially if it is received as soon as possible. Stammers are less likely to be totally eliminated in children over the age of six.

A speech and language therapist is trained to identify children whose stammers are likely to resolve naturally and which children need therapy, so early referral is key. Without adequate treatment, about 1 per cent of older children and teenagers will have developed a persistent stammer. It is estimated that 1 in every 100 adults has a stammer. There are many different speech and language therapy approaches to stammering that can help people to improve their fluency and communication skills.

If your toddler appears to have a developmental stammer, my advice would be to just give her time. Try not to pick up on the stammer or make an issue and draw attention to it, as this is likely to make the problem worse. Instead encourage your toddler to slow her speech down and let her know that you are prepared to listen.

All three of my children have had this developmental stammer as their speech and language increased. My reaction when it happened was always to say, 'Slow down. Try again,' and they would eventually get out the words that they needed to. None has been left with a permanent stammer and it had stopped by school age.

Lisps

'Lisping' is a term used to describe the way a child mispronounces words. It is very common when children are first learning to talk and something that most grow out of as their speech and language skills and pronunciation develops and matures.

If your toddler still seems to have an obvious lisp after the age of four years old, then mention it to your health visitor or GP, who may refer your child to a speech therapist.

Special words

Some toddlers have particular words for certain things you like or do and, although you know what these refer to, it's important to make any other person who cares for your toddler aware of them too. It's common for many parents and children to have different names for toilet habits – for example 'pee', 'wee', 'going for a stinky' – so this is particularly important for you to relay to nursery or pre-school staff once your toddler begins attending.

Pet names for comforters are also extremely important. *My eldest couldn't say muslin when he was very young and his word for his comfort blanket was 'mitme'. Because he called it that, my husband and I did too and the name stuck. When our second son was born and had muslin squares, my toddler called the muslins 'mitmes' and his brother automatically did the same. My daughter was born when my eldest two were eight and five years old and we all naturally referred to her muslins as her 'mitme' at bedtime too, and now that is what she calls them. When she is tired or upset, she will ask for or cry for her 'mitme'. That is not a term that any of the staff at her pre-school would know – they would never guess it means 'muslin' – so we had to make them aware of it.*

Speech stages

There are many different stages that toddlers go through as they develop their speech and language. The repetitive nature of some of them will drive you crazy but rest assured they don't last long, so try to grin and bear them until the next one comes along!

The 'What you doing?' stage

This is when you are asked by your toddler every five minutes over the course of the entire 12 hours they are awake, 'What you doing?' You can answer this question as many times as you can muster, with as many different answers as you can think of, and they will still ask you again very soon after, even though they can see and are very aware of what you are doing!

The best way I find to deal with this question when it's beginning to drive me mad is to turn it around and make it into a game and learning opportunity. When my toddler asks, 'Mummy, what you doing?' as I'm hanging the washing out, I usually say, 'I'm washing the pots.' And she will reply. 'No you not.' So I say, 'I'm cutting the grass.' And she will say, 'No you not' and I will say, 'I'm ironing.' And she will say, 'No you not.' So I say, 'Well what is Mummy doing then?' And she will immediately say what I am doing and I will praise her and say, 'See you didn't need to ask Mummy then, as you are clever and already know!' Eventually we progress to me just saying immediately in reply to her question: 'What am I doing?' and she will tell me what I'm doing.

The 'Why?' stage

After asking what you are doing repeatedly over the course of the day, the next stage is the 'why?' question. You can also answer this question as many times as you have the energy to and your toddler will still ask you 'Why?' after each answer. It generally goes something like this:

> Loren: 'Mummy, what you doing?'
> Me: 'I'm hanging the washing out.'
> Loren: 'Why?'
> Me: 'Because it needs to be dried on the washing line.'
> Loren: 'Why?'
> Me: 'Because we can't wear the clothes again until they are clean and dry.'
> Loren: 'Why?'
> Me: 'Because otherwise we would be smelly.'
> Loren: 'Why?'

You get the idea...

This is another one of those stages that will pass. Your toddler is just going through a very inquisitive stage and wants to know anything and everything she can about the environment and world she lives in. Again, you can turn the questions back to her to try and get her thinking about the possible answers. She will soon grow out of asking as she understands more about the world around her.

When to be concerned

If, by the age of three years old, your toddler still seems to have trouble understanding and following simple instructions or a period of 3–6 months has passed with no sign of language improvement, then speak to your GP or health visitor about your concerns. Equally, if you are able to understand your toddler's communication but others are not, then speech therapy may be recommended.

Have a look at the Early Years Outcomes developmental milestones in Chapter 9 for more details on the language stages children usually pass through.

More to come

Being able to finally communicate with your toddler is an exciting stage of parenting. For them and you it's much less frustrating trying to guess what it is they want or need all the time. It is your job to teach them confidence and how to express themselves in a manner that is polite and clear, so that others can understand them too. It may not be easy at times, but to watch them gradually develop their language skills is a great feeling, especially when you hear feedback from other caregivers as to how well your child communicates.

5

Learning through play

Play is essential to a child's learning and development. You can teach your child everything he needs to know before starting school, all through having fun together – from developing basic language and physical skills to learning how to be kind and caring during role-play activities.

Children love to play – they love to have fun and be happy. When they are happy and relaxed, they remember and learn things much more quickly and teaching them is much more fun for you too.

Play ideas

This chapter describes various activities and how you can use them to teach your toddler 'life skills' and basic information, such as remembering numbers, colours and letters.

Role-play

For example, dressing up, playing with dolls and teddies, setting up a train track or garage for cars. Toddlers love to mimic their parents and always want to help and be like you. During role-play activities they enjoy pretending to do the things they watch you do on a day-to-day basis. Play with

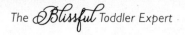

your child to begin with – show him how to do various pretend role-play and then encourage him to use teddies or dolls to mimic. He will then naturally begin to role-play without prompting.

There are, of course, a range of toys you can buy to encourage your child to role-play, but many toddlers will be just as happy, if not prefer at times, using *your* items from around the house, such as kitchen utensils, keys, old bags, shoes, and jewellery, cushions from the sofa and blankets. Once you give initial ideas the first few times, your toddler will build on this and begin to make his role-play more elaborate using these everyday items. Some popular role-play activities are:

- **Teddy bears' tea party:** Set up a blanket on the floor and have plates and cups for all the teddies and dolls involved in the tea party. Allow your toddler to have a small amount of water to serve 'tea' to the teddies. Draw pictures of food items on paper and cut them out for your toddler to use on the plates. Encourage him to hand them out to everyone at the tea party.
- **Building a den or fort:** Toddlers love hide and seek games and creating a little den or hiding place that is just for them is something they will love. Use cushions, blankets and anything else you can find to create a space for your toddler to play in. Maybe he could even take the teddy bears inside for a picnic.

Skills learned:

- Imaginative play and pretending
- How to share and play nicely with friends

- Physical skills practised while playing: gross motor skills (walking, running, jumping) and fine motor skills (picking up small objects, doing up buttons, etc)

Doing puzzles

There are so many different types of puzzles to try with your toddler, from jigsaws and shape puzzles to more complex matching games, such as Dominoes, Pairs and Picture Lotto. These games are great to play as a whole family with Mummy, Daddy and any brothers and sisters joining in too. A younger toddler will need help to learn how to play. By being on Mummy's or Daddy's team, you can provide help and encouragement and teach him how to share and enjoy games with others. These games are a great way to encourage turn-taking and will teach your toddler to be patient when playing games. This will be a tool he can take into nursery or in environments where he is with a group of children and has to share and take his turn with various toys or activities. He will have a better chance of being able to naturally make friends and get on with his peers if he's encouraged to share and be gentle and kind at home.

Skills learned:

- Uses physical skills as your toddler picks up the pieces and learns to fit them together accurately
- Encourages turn-taking and accepting help
- Develops speech as you chat about the size and shape of the puzzle pieces and how to match them together using colours or pictures

Creative play

For example, making cakes, rolling and shaping play dough, water or sand play, sticking, colouring, and painting. There are a whole host of activities you can engage your toddler in, where he learns to make thing using various materials. You can base your creative play on special occasions such as birthdays, Easter, Christmas. Encourage your child to make cards and decorations to give to people or hang up around the house. Alternatively, you can make collages and pictures to give to grandparents – they always love a bit of artwork from their grandchildren to hang on the wall or put on the fridge! Creative play is generally always coupled with mess that will need tidying and cleaning after you finish. You can limit the amount of mess by laying down an old plastic sheet or an old blanket or duvet cover on the floor and using newspaper or a plastic table cloth on the table. Put your toddler in old clothes that you don't mind getting dirty when you engage in a creative activity. If he's worried about getting his clothes dirty, he won't be so enthusiastic and want to get as involved. You could also buy a painting apron for him or use an old shirt over his clothes to protect them.

Skills learned:

- Painting, drawing, playing with sand and water, and various other arts and crafts, all help to develop fine motor skills in toddlers, which will in turn aid their pencil control, so they are ready to begin writing with more accuracy by the time they begin school.
- As well as using various physical skills, like their fine motor skills, as they pick items up and make their creation, this is another opportunity to chat about the colours and shapes

Tuff spot

A tuff spot is a large plastic tray that builders use for mixing sand and cement and other building materials and can be purchased from a DIY store. However, they are proving very popular among parents as they are a great place to allow your toddler to engage in messy play, without your house or garden ending up messy too!

There are literally hundreds of ideas and materials you could put into the tuff spot, along with small world toys, cars, utensils, etc., to allow your child to explore and do what most toddlers love to do – get messy!

You can even have a big bowl of soapy water outside for your toddler to get straight into when he has had enough and wants to wash off all that messy-play gunk. If the weather isn't so good, then the tuff spot can also be used indoors – just place some large towels or blankets down and then the tuff spot on top to save your floor from becoming dirty.

Using various materials and toys in the tuff spot gives you great opportunities to develop your toddler's language as well as physical and imaginative skills, as you talk while he plays about shape, size and texture, etc. This is an activity you can plan to do with a friend's child, so they can enjoy it together or even with you, the parent.

of things and stimulate and broaden your toddler's intellect. You can ask him questions about the materials he's using – how strong they are, how he can adapt his ideas to change something he has created into something else and predict what may happen if he does certain things. There is a great deal of concentration needed, too, when being creative and encouraging this from an early age will enable your toddler to continue to think about how to solve problems as he gets older too, much more easily.

- Counting can also be incorporated into any of these activities and various maths skills taught – more or less and bigger and smaller, for example.

- Social and emotional development: Creative play is a great way for children to express themselves. It can also be a way to encourage a very shy child to socialise with others as he talks about what he is making or how, for example, the sand, water or play dough feels as he touches it. As he gains confidence, he can begin to create things with his peers and they will help each other along the way.

TIP

It's fun to tune into your inner child and allow yourself to get messy on occasion too! Your toddler will really appreciate his usually restrained, like-to-be clean Mummy, engaging in such a fun activity!

Outdoor play

Your toddler will love outdoor activities, such as jumping on a trampoline, riding bikes and scooters, going to the park, running around and climbing. Be there to support and praise your toddler to encourage his independence and build his confidence. Once he has completed a physical challenge, he will be more confident and want to do it again. Repeating it will mean he gets better at it and continue to push himself to do new physical challenges.

These outdoor activities all encourage use of your child's physical skills and this is just as important as teaching him how to count, write or learn his colours. He needs to practise walking, running, climbing and balancing to get better at them. Some children are naturally very active and want to climb and prefer physical activity to engaging in things that require mental concentration.

TIP

I know it's worrying when toddlers are learning new physical skills, such as climbing and balancing. It's natural to be concerned that they will fall and get hurt. Any doubt and anxiety you have will rub off on your toddler, though, so try to be positive and believe in him. It will influence how he tackles new challenges.

Outdoor play is also a good way to teach your toddler about the environment and the world we live in. Children are very inquisitive and love to ask questions and learn new things, so use this enthusiasm to teach him about animals, plants, trees and how to keep the environment clean and tidy for the animals that live in it. You could go on walks and make a nature trail with a list of things you want your toddler to look out for and help him tick them off as he sees them.

Reading books

Reading is a lovely activity to do with your toddler to calm or wind him down. It gives you a one-to-one special time together and he will enjoy the individual attention he gets.

I always try to do 10 minutes of reading time before bed with all three of my children individually. They all love having me to themselves for that short period of time, without siblings around, and it's nice for me to be able to truly listen to them talk about their day, without the distractions of others interrupting. It's a lovely activity to do together before bed as part of your evening routine.

Encouraging your toddler to enjoy books with you and reading alone from a young age has huge benefits for speech and language development. Listening to you read and hearing a range of words and the intonation you use as you read him stories, will in turn help him to use expression in his speech and develop more personality to put into the conversations he has. Continuing to read to him as he gets older will also help him learn to add more expression as he learns to read to you and be more adventurous with the words he uses in his writing at school.

Reading a book together is also an activity you can suggest to your toddler if you need to calm him down a little. It's also a useful way to give him your attention during feeding time with a younger sibling.

Singing songs and dancing

All toddlers love to sing and dance, whether it be to nursery rhymes or music that's on the TV or radio. Your toddler will love you joining in with him and it's a great way to bond and have some fun if you are feeling a bit stressed. Teaching your toddler various songs and nursery rhymes will help to improve his memory – he will begin to remember the words and actions to the songs you sing. It will also develop and extend the language he uses on a day-to-day basis, teaching him new words. Nursery rhymes CDs are fun to listen to at home and in the car,

Hide and seek

This is a game most toddlers love to play but they need practice at it to learn the art of keeping quiet in their chosen hiding place, without jumping up and revealing themselves or talking.

We enjoy playing this as a family with one of us staying with our toddler and having the job of hiding her before we hide ourselves. Now she's three years old she has got the hang of the game quite well and will sit quietly until she is found. However, when we first began playing it with her, she would call my older boys and be so noisy they easily knew where she was. They were great at playing along with the game, though, and looking in various places first declaring, 'No, she's not there,' before finally finding her.

Now we try to make the game a little more interesting, particularly if the boys are hiding in a less obvious place and our toddler daughter is getting a little despondent with being unable to find them easily. We ask the hidden people to make an animal noise from the place that they are hiding in to help our toddler find them more easily. It's pretty funny to hear my little girl shouting, 'Bark like a dog, Ollie,' and then hearing a 'woof woof' noise come from the nearest cupboard. It certainly makes the game more interesting and fun for everyone!

or you could play the soundtrack from your toddler's favourite film. Apps can be downloaded for a tablet to teach your toddler various songs and dancing and there are many interactive books that play songs and are fun to read and sing along to together.

You can even make up your own songs to help him learn various things. When I'm counting with my toddler, I tend to do it in a sing-song voice. She enjoys hearing me do it and tries to repeat it back. It means I can easily get her to repeat 1, 2, 3, 4, 5 back to me 10 or more times quite happily. By the time she has repeated it a few times, she remembers the number order without even realising she is being taught something important!

Small world toys

This is play equipment that is set up to replicate an activity or job or role that happens in real life. It offers special learning opportunities as children try to mimic what they have seen and they can act out different play activities.

All areas of a toddler's development are used and challenged during small world play. This is a great activity to do with your toddler and really get his imagination working by talking about going to different places using the cars or trains, or by testing his memory skills on places you have been together as a family. Small world toys are used regularly in childcare settings, so it's good to get your toddler used to playing with these types of toys, particularly when you have friends round to play, as this will be another opportunity to encourage sharing. Toys that are used for small world activities include:

- Trains and train track
- Doll's house with dolls and furniture
- Cars and garage
- Animals: a farmyard or zoo

Bathtime fun

Making bathtime a fun experience will help to relax your toddler if he has any fears of water or even hair-washing, and is a positive way to end the day and start the bedtime routine.

There are many different bath toys you can buy, but you don't need to spend a fortune as most toddlers will be happy with empty household containers. Bathtime games include filling and pouring, testing which items sink or float, playing pretend games with bath toys and even singing. There will inevitably be a mess – it's usually a sign that bathtime has been a fun experience. Try not to stress about it, though, or make your toddler feel like he's not allowed to splash or make a mess – this will add stress to what should be a fun experience.

Types of play

At different stages between the ages of 2–4 years, your toddler will engage in different types of play in social situations. Playing games with him at home and encouraging turn-taking with you, Daddy and siblings will help him understand how to play with his friends.

Parallel play

When two toddlers are playing with the same toys – for example, cars or dolls – but not actually playing or engaging with each other it is known as parallel play. They are each involved in their own imaginative play. They may observe and imitate but won't interact. Parallel play is usually first observed in children aged 2–3 years. The older they get, the less frequently they will engage in this type of play because they gain confidence and make friends who they interact with during play.

Solitary (independent) play

Playing alone is usually associated with babies and younger toddlers. However, there may be occasions where older toddlers and pre-school children occasionally engage in independent play, particularly in new environments or if they are tired and not feeling very sociable.

TIP

Although it is fun and very important to play with your toddler to aid his development and teach him new things, it is also important that he is happy to play independently. This will help his confidence when it's time to start pre-school or nursery, and mean he's less likely to find the transition difficult.

Imitative or associative play

This is when your toddler and another child copy each other. For example, one child throws himself on the floor in a silly way and the other copies, or one jumps, so the other jumps too. Your toddler may also copy you – if you are mixing something while cooking, he may want his own bowl and spoon to mix. In this type of play, children begin to interact with each other by talking, taking turns with toys and copying, but each child acts alone rather than helping each other complete any one task.

Co-operative play

As they get older, usually over three years, most toddlers begin to want to play with other children. Your toddler may offer toys or say something to try to engage another toddler to play, and he will happily wander off and help a child build something or share toys within a small world set-up. He is likely to start chatting to his playmates, too.

By the end of his toddler years, you would hope that your child is:

- Happy to share and interact with his peers
- Talking to others when trying to solve a particular challenge
- Able to take direction from other children who give advice as they play and engage in an activity

Your toddler will develop and begin to want to play with others as he gets older as long as you encourage his confidence and independence. Of course there are always going to be times when he would like you to play with him and be involved in what he's doing, and also times where he wants to engage in solitary play. That is fine and perfectly normal. Sometimes we all need a bit of alone time without interaction from others. As long as you teach your toddler the basic social skills of sharing and caring behaviour, he will continue to develop his confidence and independence through the everyday play activities you and other child carers provide.

6
Toilet training

Many parents dread this part of a child's development as there seems to be so much pressure from friends and family members, all imparting their wisdom and tips about how they toilet trained their own children. When someone is telling you that you should do certain things in a certain way at a certain time, remember each child is different and each family is different. If toilet training is done at the right time, when a child is ready, then it doesn't have to be a stressful experience for anyone. Yes, there will be accidents to begin with, but as long as you are prepared for those and react in the right way, your toddler will soon get the hang of learning when she needs to go to the toilet and telling you in good time.

When should you start toilet training?
There is no right or wrong age to begin toilet training your toddler. What you are looking for are *signs* that your toddler is ready to begin the first stages of toilet training. There are various behavioural, physical and cognitive signs to look for, listed below.

Behavioural signs

Your toddler:

- Knows *before* she is doing a poo and wanders off to hide to do it in her nappy or crouches down and does it and then tells you before, afterwards, or admits to it when you ask her
- Can pull her trousers up and down herself
- Shows signs of independence like wanting to do things for herself without your help
- Will sit down quietly and concentrate for a few minutes at a time
- Doesn't like the feeling of wearing her nappy when it is wet or soiled
- Is interested in the idea of using the toilet – she watches you and wants to try on underwear
- Is in a co-operative stage of her development and not a resistant one

Cognitive signs

Your toddler:

- Can understand simple instructions, such as 'Go and put that in the bin'
- Understands what wee and poo is and has words she uses for them
- Shows physical awareness that she needs to do, or is doing, a wee or poo

Physical signs

Your toddler:

- Has a dry nappy on regular occasions when waking from a daytime nap – this shows that her bladder is developed enough to hold urine for a length of time
- Can walk steadily and even run

> **TIP**
>
> *Don't be pressured by family members and friends comparing their toddlers to yours, even if they are the same age. All children are different, even among siblings, and will all be ready at different times. If you rush toilet training and begin before your toddler is ready, it won't work as well as it could do and will be a much more stressful process than it needs to be for both of you. This will make regression more likely to occur.*

Twins

It's very unlikely that twins will be ready to be toilet trained at exactly the same time. In my experience, one twin is always ready before the other. It is better to toilet train them separately rather than trying to train the second twin before the signs of readiness (see above) are there. Training twins at the same time when one isn't quite ready is more likely to cause issues for both. The twin that isn't ready will have accidents and struggle, and the twin that was ready will not like all the attention the other twin is getting. This is likely to cause regression and make the whole process more difficult than it needs to be because you are unable to give them the attention they need to succeed. The twin who isn't initially ready will be encouraged by their sibling anyway and when you are ready to begin that toilet training, the process will be much easier.

Toilet or potty?

Some experts will recommend you toilet train straight to the toilet rather than the potty, to save another transition later on. In my experience this is a totally personal choice between

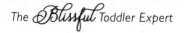

parent and child, and environmental factors, as described below, can also affect your decision.

If you don't have a downstairs toilet, training directly to the toilet will be more difficult. In the first few days and weeks of potty training, when your toddler tells you that she needs to wee, you have around 10–20 seconds maximum to get her somewhere to do it! If you have to make your way to an upstairs toilet, then by the time you get there, even if you carry her, it may just be too late and she will have wet herself. After a few days of this happening your toddler may get despondent and frustrated at the whole process, even though she's doing everything she can to get to the toilet in time.

Of course if you persevere then eventually things will improve but if you don't have a downstairs toilet then it may be better to use the potty to begin with until your toddler's bladder control improves.

I have used the potty with my three children when beginning potty training and combined this with using a booster seat and step for the toilet too. None of my children or any of the toddlers I toilet trained while working as a nanny, nor any of the parents I have advised, have had any problems with their toddler transitioning from using a potty to going on the toilet.

How to potty train
Approach potty training in stages to gradually introduce the idea to your toddler.

Stage 1
Have a potty in the house – maybe in the upstairs bathroom – so your toddler can get used to the idea of it. Read books about sitting on the toilet/potty as part of a bedtime routine.

Don't read them every night, of course, but every now and then as a build-up to the idea of potty training.

Stage 2

Talk about your own toilet needs! I'm sure your toddler has followed you to the toilet since she could walk or even crawl. Now isn't the time to be shy! Going for a wee or poo needs to be discussed constantly so that your child sees it as a normal thing – for Mummy, Daddy and any siblings. If you are going to the toilet, say to your toddler, 'Mummy is just going for a wee wee.'

As she follows you, which let's be fair is pretty inevitable, talk her through the process as you are doing it. I always try to make it sound interesting: 'Oh, can you listen for Mummy's wee wee?' Then once it starts: 'Here it comes! Clever girl, Mummy!' By getting your toddler to praise you and watch what you do, she will get into the habit of learning that's what she will eventually do. Get some tissue and explain to her what you are doing: 'Mummy needs to wipe so she is not all wet, then put the paper in the toilet. Now I'm going to pull my knickers and trousers up and flush the toilet. Say bye bye to the wee wee. Right now Mummy needs to wash her hands.' Then talk her through the whole process of handwashing. Repeat the same if you need to do a poo as well.

It's important that you go through this with your toddler, so she sees it all as normal.

Send her to the toilet with Daddy, too. It's important she sees that you both do the same routine even if Daddy wees in a different way. You can progress to talking about the basic differences between boys and girls. My toddler loves going through every one she knows and telling me if they have a willy. Even at this young age, she understands that the boys all have a willy and that girls don't. She also understands that Daddy and her brothers stand up to go to the toilet but she sits down like Mummy because we are girls.

Once your toddler is beginning to grasp stage 2, you can progress to stage 3.

Stage 3

Encourage your toddler to begin sitting on the potty at bathtime. Take all her clothes off ready for the bath and ask her each night if she would like to sit on it before she gets in the bath. You can tie it in with you sitting on the toilet (even if you don't actually need to go!) 'Look Mummy is going to have a wee wee on the toilet. Do you want to sit on your potty and try for a wee wee?'

If she doesn't want to, then don't push it. Once you get off the toilet, then you could offer to read her a book while she's on the potty to see if that encourages her. If she does want you to read the book, then talk to her at the same time. At the end you can say, 'Right let's get up and see if there are any wee wees?' If there are none, then just say, 'No wee wee? Never mind, you are a good girl for sitting on the potty!' Then high five or cuddle her, with praise.

Obviously if your toddler does on a rare occasion do a wee, then you need to make a big fuss! Tell her how clever she is and then get her to help you empty the wee from the potty into the toilet! Again, give her lots of praise.

Do this sitting on the potty or toilet before bathtime for a week or two before moving on to stage 4. If you want to encourage your toddler to sit on the potty at other times too, such as first thing in the morning or when waking from a nap, then you can do, but in my experience, bathtime seems to be the easiest and least stressful time of the day to try it.

Stage 4

It's time for a shopping trip! Go out with your toddler and choose some pants for her to wear a day or two before you plan to start toilet training properly. I would recommend you buy at least 30 pairs. It may sound a lot but by the time you have had a few wet pairs in the first few days and they have to go through the wash and dry cycle, you will be grateful for that many.

Character underwear is good if your child has a particular favourite. Also buy some special stickers for her star chart: animal or character ones work well as she will enjoy choosing a different one each time. Alternatively, use coloured stars. Initially I wouldn't use a pull-up on your toddler during the day if you are going to be at home. You only need to consider using them if you know your child will have to be in the car for a long period of time or you will be in an environment where it will be difficult to get to a toilet fast.

The night before you are planning to put your toddler in pants, explain what you are going to do: 'When you wake up in the morning, we are going to put your big girl knickers on.'

Stage 5

When your toddler wakes in the morning, it is best to take her nappy off straight away and encourage her to choose a pair of pants to put on for the first time. Encourage her to sit on the potty or toilet before she puts the pants on to try for a wee wee. Give her lots of praise for sitting on there, even if she doesn't actually do anything. Remind her that she needs to tell you when she needs a wee wee or poo poo and then you can help her sit on the potty or toilet. You can ask or encourage her to sit on the toilet or potty a little while after she has had a drink. See below for more directions on this.

TIP

Try to allow your toddler just to roam around the house in her pants and a top rather than putting trousers on too for the first few days. If she has too many layers that feel heavy around her bottom, then she may feel like she is still wearing a nappy. Obviously when you go out you will have to put trousers on her. Try to stick to loose-fitting cotton ones or if it's summer time then a skirt or loose-fitting shorts that are easy for her to pull up and down.

If you have older children to walk or drive to school, then it may be worth trying to get your partner or a friend to collect and drop them off for the first day or two of potty training.

I recommended setting aside the first three days to stay home and establish the basics of potty training to give it the best chance of working. This is more of a difficult task if both parents work, so it is helpful to wait until you have a run of two or three days at home – maybe on a long weekend or when you have some annual leave and can really focus your attention on toilet training. I've found it helpful to have a piece of paper and pen handy to keep a note of the times you give your toddler a drink and when she wees on the potty, when she has accidents, etc. It's good to note roughly how long after a small drink that she needs to wee. That way you can work out a rough pattern and look for the first signs she needs a wee. In my experience toddlers usually need a wee roughly 20–30 minutes after a drink in these early stages of potty training. If you have noted drink times, then you will be able to work out when to encourage her to sit on the potty or toilet.

Have lots of books and toys to play with so you can base yourself in one room for the first day. Your toddler is bound to have accidents, and she needs to have them to experience that wet feeling so that she can attempt to ask for the potty or toilet before things get to that stage next time. Even if she does begin to wee in her pants, or seem to have done it all on the floor, still encourage her to sit on the potty or toilet afterwards to see if there is any more wee wee. Give lots of praise when she does this, then put clean pants on her.

It's important not to make your toddler feel bad for weeing her pants. It's a new learning experience and learning to use the potty or toilet won't happen immediately. Write down all the good catches in the toilet or potty, when she's asked to use the potty or toilet, and when she's had accidents. By the end of the first day it's highly likely you will have had more accidents than catches, but that is perfectly normal and as long as you have had two or three successful wees in the potty it is progress you can work on.

Don't forget to use the special chart and let her put a sticker on each time she does a wee or poo in the potty.

Stage 6

By day 3–4 of toilet training, your toddler should be beginning to have more wees on the potty than misses. If you are still mainly the instigator of when she sits on the potty by encouraging her based on when she last had a drink, take a little step back and encourage her to take the lead in asking for the potty or toilet. She needs to learn to recognise the feeling she gets just before her wee comes and ask to go accordingly. She will never do that if you always sit her on the potty or toilet.

She may have a few accidents the first few times but just remind her that she needs to ask you. You can ask her if she needs a wee roughly 20–30 minutes after a drink but if she says no, then go with it and don't pressure her to sit on there if she insists she doesn't need to go. If she does have an accident, then change her as directed and remind her that she needs to tell you when she needs a wee and she can have a sticker for being so clever.

Continue to write down at roughly what point she needs to wee after a drink. That will give you an idea of when you need to be aware of her wanting to wee. Over the days and weeks after you begin toilet training, her bladder control will increase and she won't need to go so often. Again you will notice a rough pattern and realise that you have a little more time to make it to the toilet than you did in the beginning.

Pull-ups and nappies

You will still need to use pull-up nappies on your toddler at night-time and for any day naps she may still have. Some toddlers aren't keen on having a nappy back on again, even for naps. I always explain it by saying to them that when they are sleeping their willy or bottom is sleeping too so they need to wear a nappy until it's time to wake up. Once your toddler wakes, take her nappy or pull-up off straight away and encourage her to sit on the potty or toilet, particularly if the nappy is still dry.

Some people will tell you that you shouldn't use pull-ups at any other time than for naps. In an ideal world I would agree with that and if you are potty training your first child and can base yourself at home quite a lot until toilet training is established, then it's quite possible you won't have the need to use pull-ups at all.

I didn't use pull-ups at all except for nap/sleep times when toilet training my first two children. However, when I reached the time to begin toilet training my third child it was not as easy to base myself at home with her for a week or two to concentrate fully on toilet training. We had school runs to do, after-school clubs to take her brothers to and hanging around at the sides of football pitches and swimming lessons! There wasn't always a toilet as close by as she or I would have liked so we needed the use of a pull-up to prevent having countless outfit changes!

The times that I did put a pull-up on her when we were out and about, I would always remind her as I put it on that she still needed to tell me when she needed to use the toilet.

She did always ask and never used it like a nappy to just wee in whenever she felt like it. However, having the pull-up on gave me the security that I wouldn't be 'caught out' and have her wee herself at the most inconvenient time. The pull-up bought us time on occasions if the toilet wasn't close by.

She always did her best to hold her wee while we rushed to find a toilet, but inevitably there were times in the first few weeks of toilet training that she would have started the wee by the time I got her to the toilet. She would always finish it on the toilet, though, and never used the pull-up to do her wee in without asking for the toilet first.

Toilet or potty?

None of my children or any of the ones I have trained while working as a nanny, in a nursery or whose parents I have advised, have ever been bothered about whether they use the potty or toilet. I encourage parents to use a mixture of both from the beginning. The potty is helpful for the first few days and although I did always take the potty out with me, more often than not children are happy to use the toilet. The novelty of it is exciting for most children, especially if they see you use it first and you encourage and praise them enthusiastically.

It's a good idea to take the potty out with you for the first few times, though, as there may be occasions where the potty is preferable — for example, if the toilet environment is not a very clean or hygienic one! (Some public toilets at outdoor playgrounds can be a bit smelly and not a place where you would like your child to sit her little bottom!)

Poo is special

It is *very* normal for the poo side of toilet training to take much longer than the wee side, despite the fact that your toddler has been showing signs of knowing she is about to do a poo in her nappy for months before you begin toilet training. You may have noticed that she has been wandering off and hiding in the corner when she needs to poo and then reappearing with a smell wafting around her so that you know she has done it.

However, doing a poo in her nappy secretly and then having her nappy changed and you taking it away and throwing it in the bin means she has probably never even seen what her poo looks like! Coupled with the fact that you have probably (very innocently) been saying jokingly to her every time since she was a baby, 'Ewww yuk, poo, poo. Are you stinky?' or something similar. This will mean that her association with poo has been a very negative one from an early age and not something she will want to see or get excited about as she begins potty training.

I have found the best way to get a toddler used to and happy about the idea of doing a poo somewhere other than her nappy is to work very hard on stage 2 (see page 161), before you even attempt to start toilet training. Take her to the toilet with you. Tell her before you go that you need a poo, 'Quick Mummy needs a poo poo, quick let's go to the toilet.' Talk her through the whole process of *you* doing a poo on the toilet, wiping your bottom and looking at the poo in the toilet before you flush it away. Make sure you do *not* use negative words, such as, 'That's yucky' or 'disgusting.' You can talk about the size, 'Wow Mummy has done a big poo poo', etc., and then ask her to help you flush it away and say bye bye to the poo poo. By doing all of this she will begin to think of going for a poo as a very normal routine thing and her fear of it will lessen.

You can then talk her through the handwashing and get her to praise you for being a clever girl and doing the poo in the toilet. Daddy can also go through this process and I'm sure your toddler will even follow siblings into the bathroom. No room for being shy with a toddler in the house! I usually have the toddler and the dog follow me into the bathroom and one of the boys calling asking where I am all at the same time! I can't remember the last time I went to the toilet in peace! Ha ha.

Getting your toddler to do that first poo on the potty will be the milestone that makes her realise that she can do it in a place other than her nappy, and your reaction to it will be crucial.

Give her lots of praise, high fives and a special sticker on her chart for a poo in the toilet or potty. Let her help you empty it into the toilet or say bye bye to it if she does it on the toilet, then flush it away and wash her hands.

You need to be very 'on the ball' in the first days and weeks to notice the first signs of your toddler needing to poo and encourage her towards the toilet. Your toddler may have certain signs that you recognise – wandering off and hiding, crouching down, bending over, or a particular facial expression as she begins to poo. Some may even have a certain time of the day that they always tend to do a poo, so you can be particularly vigilant at this time.

With my toddlers as soon as I noticed these first few signs I would say, 'Do you need a poo? Quick, quick, let's go to the potty/toilet.' You don't have much time to play with once a toddler begins to poo and that's sometimes why it takes a bit longer to achieve poos on the toilet *all* the time. If you are not in the same room as your toddler all the time, then you may miss that cue and by the time you have noticed it's too late and the poo has already been done in her pants.

Rush her off to the toilet before she gets time to think about it, praising her all the time. Reassure her as she is sitting on the toilet or potty as she may be very scared about the idea of doing the poo and having to see it after. If she doesn't want to look at it, that's fine. The more poos she does on the toilet or potty, the less scared she will be by the whole process.

Give massive praise if she manages it – compare her to you and Daddy or older siblings: 'Wow, you are so so clever! You did a poo in the toilet like Mummy, Daddy and Jack! Let's go tell Daddy!' Offer stickers or some sort of reward that may encourage her to try to get the poo in the toilet again next time. Once she has managed to poo two or three times in the toilet, her confidence will grow and she will not be so scared next time.

CASE STUDY: Martha and Helen

Helen contacted me to ask for advice about her daughter Martha, who was her third child. She had toilet trained very easily, managing to do lots of successful wees on the potty and toilet. However, the poo side of things was not improving and Martha had got to the point where she was holding it all day while wearing knickers. However, when she was asleep at night and not able to hold it in any more, as her bowels relaxed, she would end up soiling herself and the bed in the middle of the night. These words are from Martha's mother Helen:

'There's no age at which I start potty training. It's more about intuition and speech development. Martha was just under two-and-a-half when we started but was really good in terms of speech and development. She was terrified of the potty to start with, which I hadn't experienced with my older two boys, so we made a "magic" potty that entailed about £5 worth of fairy stickers put on every available space. Peeing went well. Obviously there was the odd accident, which is to be expected, but we did the songs and dance and praise stuff and it was relatively easy and she was even dry at night, but the girl would not poop!

All would go well, she'd get up in the morning and pee on the potty, and would be fine until around lunchtime, then she'd go and hide behind a chair/beneath a table/in the shed… then you'd smell her! She wasn't frightened of pooping. She was frightened of doing it on a potty. After about a fortnight of this and the final straw being that she started holding it and pooping her PJs at 3am, I emailed Lisa and she told me to take Martha to the loo with me and try to make the whole idea of going to the toilet a normal experience that she could relate to.

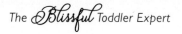

I must say it was initially very uncomfortable sitting on the loo with a two-year-old coaching me! But I held her hand and told her, "Look, see, Mummy can do it. You can too. Nothing to be scared of ..." That helped so much and was the turning point for her. We had maybe one or two close calls, but other than that never had a poop in the pants again. Before I spoke to Lisa I was getting increasingly cross and it wasn't helping the situation but it was so frustrating as she knew exactly what she was doing, which frustrated me even more! Lisa's advice helped me take a fresh look at the situation and understand what Martha might be feeling and as soon as I relaxed and used lots of positive praise to help her fears, she quickly settled down and wasn't scared of doing a poo on the potty any more.'

Learning to wipe their own bottom

When your toddler does begin doing regular poos on the toilet and learns to go to the toilet alone, encourage her to always call you to wipe her bottom. You can explain what you are doing – that you need to keep wiping her until there is no more poo poo on the tissue and that means it is finally clean and she can pull her knickers up.

Pre-schools and nurseries are happy to continue this, but you will need to teach your toddler how to wipe her own bottom by the time she starts primary school at the age of four years. Have a few practice sessions at home where you get her to wipe her own bottom and check it once she's finished. Encourage her to wipe some more if needed.

You may have a few occasions when your toddler first starts school where you need to do an extra clean-up when she gets home, as she hasn't quite managed to wipe her bottom well enough. Just be aware of this and some extra bum-wiping practice sessions at home may be needed. Moist toilet wipes are great to have at home – encourage your toddler to use them to ensure their bottom is clean after doing a poo. Again, praise and positive encouragement is the key and no negative words to make her feel like she's not doing a good enough job.

Constipation

Some toddlers can become constipated due to the fact that they try to hold their poo all day until they have their bedtime nappy on. They also may try holding it indefinitely through fear of going. Eventually it has to come though no matter how good they are at holding it, and for most it tends to be late in the evening or even in the middle of the night when their bowel is most relaxed and they are too tired to hold it any more.

A 3am poo is no fun for anyone, but if this is a regular occurrence then it is a sign that your toddler is holding her poo during the day so she doesn't have to deal with it, especially if, so far, she hasn't got into the habit of doing a regular one on the toilet or potty.

Try to ensure your toddler has a good amount of fibre in her diet to prevent constipation caused this way, but equally avoid fibre and meat late in the day or evening as that is likely to cause a poo overnight or disturb sleep in the early mornings. If your toddler prefers to ask for a nappy to do her poo in during the beginning stages of toilet training it's fine – most parents would find that preferable to cleaning pants with poo in.

When you do take the nappy off containing poo, then show it to her and don't use words like yuk, smelly, disgusting, or dirty. If it is a hard lump and easy to put in the toilet then that would be a good thing to do with her as a transition stage, which she can help you with. Say something like, 'Wow, that's a big poo poo. Can you come and help Mummy put it in the toilet and we will flush it away.' Put it in the loo and then encourage her to say, 'Bye bye poo poo.'

As your toddler becomes more confident with this process, she won't be so scared and you can begin to encourage her to do the poo directly on the toilet.

Dealing with accidents

It's very important that you don't tell your toddler off if she does wee or even poo her knickers. You can reiterate that next time she should tell you when she needs a wee or poo without making her feel bad for not making it this time. Say something like: 'Oh dear, never mind. Let's get you some dry pants. Let's go and try for more wee or poo on the toilet and then Mummy will put some dry pants on you. Where do wee wees and poo poos go? [hopefully she will answer the toilet or potty] Yes, that's right – we don't do them in our pants, do we? Where does Mummy do her wee wee? [answers] Yes, that's right. Can you tell Mummy when you need a wee or poo and then we can sit you on the toilet or potty. Yes? Good girl.'

Of course, there will be times that your toddler will wet or poo herself at the most inconvenient time ever – my daughter usually did this once we all had coats and shoes on and were ready to rush out the door to do the school run for her brothers. Suddenly a big puddle would appear on the floor as I was rounding her brothers up with their bags, etc. I knew that it was probably my fault as I was so rushed dealing with her brothers that she hadn't been able to tell me in time and wet herself before getting to the potty or toilet.

It makes for a very stressful situation though and shouting at her or telling your toddler off for making you even later is not going to change the current situation you find yourself in.

In fact, it's more likely to make her regress with toilet training as the stress and pressure will be too much for her to cope with.

Regression

There are various situations and events that may make your toddler likely to regress with toilet training.

New baby

I always advise parents *against* beginning toilet training unless you have a good 3–6 months to get it established before a new baby arrives. Even then it's likely that you still may have the odd accident once the baby arrives. That's very normal and your toddler is just showing signs of being a little insecure by the whole arrival of a new person to the family unit. Reassure her and try to make some extra special time to spend with her and she will soon settle down. Introduce a star or sticker chart with rewards to give her motivation and make her feel special.

Starting nursery/moving house

Again these are two big life changes to the daily routine that can cause toilet regression. Reassuring your toddler and continuing to praise and reward the times she does make it to the toilet on time will soon get her back on track again. If you have stopped using a sticker/star chart as she had been doing very well, it may be worth re-introducing it with some exciting new stickers. That will help her head back in the right direction again.

Illness

If your child becomes ill with a virus or cold, it can sometimes make her regress and begin to have more toileting accidents as she just doesn't have the energy to tell you when she needs to go to the loo. I've found using a pull-up during these times can help. Still encourage your toddler to tell you when she needs the toilet but as she will tend to doze in and out of sleep a lot when ill, it's easier to leave a pull-up on her rather than putting one on then taking it off constantly each time she falls asleep. It's usually very easy to get toddlers back on track again when they are feeling better and motivated to please.

Toilet seats

Some toddlers worry about the size of a toilet and falling down it. You can buy a special toddler seat that fits over the top of your normal toilet seat that makes the hole smaller. When toddlers sit on it, they feel much more secure and know they won't fall down. You can also buy a small step that toddlers can stand on to get up on to the seat. It can also be used to reach the sink for handwashing. Both of these can be bought from most supermarkets and baby and childcare superstores.

Boys

Many parents ask me if they should expect their toddler boy to stand up at the toilet as soon as they begin potty training. My advice is always to be guided by him and when he is ready.

His height can sometimes be a big deciding factor. I've generally found that boys are usually keen to stand up at the toilet when they are tall enough to lean up against it and their willy can just rest over the side of the pan and pee into the toilet. It will take some practice for him to get his aim right. Encourage him to give his willy a little shake after he has done a wee to get all the drips off and prevent him getting a sore willy with it being wet and moist in his pants.

TIP

A good way to encourage your son to wee in the right direction into the toilet is to place a coloured bouncy ball or something similar in there and get him to aim his wee towards it and try to hit it. This makes the whole experience more fun for him to do and if he enjoys the idea of trying to hit the bouncy ball, then he's more likely to tell you when he needs a wee to go and try it each time, rather than wee himself.

Once his aim improves you can progress to using a piece of toilet paper in the loo and get him to aim at that instead. You can do this to begin with if you don't want to be putting bouncy balls or anything else down the toilet and then fishing them out, but of course it won't be as much fun for him!

Girls

Toddler girls need to be encouraged to wipe their front bottom after doing a wee on the toilet or potty to prevent them becoming sore. Teach your daughter to wipe from front to back, rather than back to front. This is to prevent bacteria from her anus being bought forward to her front bottom.

When to give up

There has to be a point where you say enough is enough and admit that toilet training doesn't seem to be working and your child is just not ready at this moment in time, or because of circumstances. The instances where it may be necessary to

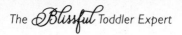

put your toddler back in nappies or pull-ups full time are as follows:

- You are 2–3 weeks into the potty training process and your toddler is still not asking to use the potty or toilet at all, has lots of accidents in her pants on a daily basis and shows no enthusiasm for wanting to ask to go. She may not be bothered about working towards any reward for using the potty or toilet and happily wear wet pants without telling you she has even done anything.

- Illness or a major routine change can cause regression even if your toddler seemed to have grasped toilet training and was having barely any accidents. If she regresses badly and you are unable to get her back on track using the earlier advice of praise, reward and sticker charts and the daily toilet training is a big stress for both of you that doesn't seem to be improving, it is time to back off. If you put her back in nappies for a few weeks and then go right back to stage 1, and take things slowly, then it will be much easier to toilet train her at a time when she is ready.

Night-time nappy and being dry at night

It varies as to when toddlers are ready to stop wearing a nappy or pull-up at night-time and it isn't always at the same time as they become dry during the day. It's worth remembering that many children aged 3–4 years old still need a night-time nappy and bedwetting is considered very normal up to the age of 5. Also 1 in 6 five-year-olds still wet the bed occasionally or regularly. Signs to look for:

- Her naptime nappy is always dry when she wakes up and she is not desperate for a wee as soon as she wakes
- Her night-time nappy is sometimes dry when she wakes in the morning
- Her night-time nappy is still warm when you take it off in the morning – this means she is doing the wee contained in it as soon as she wakes in the morning rather than in the night

To help your toddler to stop wearing nappies at night-time:

- Reduce and stop all drinks an hour before bedtime
- Encourage her to have a wee right before you put her bedtime nappy on so that she has an empty bladder as she goes to bed

---

Lifting

Some parents wake their toddler at night before they go to bed and sit them on the toilet to prevent night-time bedwetting. This is called 'lifting'. You need to ensure that your child is fully awake and understands what you are doing, rather than being sat on the toilet half asleep.

TIP

Once you begin to attempt night-time training, it's a good idea to buy a waterproof mattress protector to put under the bed sheet. You can also buy disposable bed mats that are absorbent. These can be bought from the supermarket in the nappy aisle.

My children were all toilet trained very differently, both during the day and at night. My eldest was around 21 months when he began showing all the signs of being ready to begin toilet training. We went through all of the early stages and when he was 22 months, I began potty training him. He had the wee side cracked in a week and the poo side took him around a month to get the hang of fully. As he gradually grasped the idea, we had quite a few instances of him wandering into a corner to hide and do the poo in his pants. As soon as he was dry during the day, he didn't want to wear a nappy at night either. We had already transitioned him from a cot to a bed because he went through a stage of launching himself out of the cot repeatedly over a period of days, so we decided it was safer to move him to a bed. Once I had put him to bed, he would take the nappy off and leave it on the floor. After a few nights of this, replacing his nappy while he was asleep and then him taking it off again after we had gone to bed, I realised we needed to change tactics. I placed a potty in his room and told him if he needed a wee then he should get up and do it on the potty, then get back in bed and in the morning we would empty any wees into the toilet. Thankfully this worked and we never had a wet bed after that. He was dry day and night by just over two years old.

My second son's speech was not as developed as his brother's, so I waited a little longer before toilet training him. At age two-and-a-half, he tried a pair of his brother's pants on one day insisting I take his nappy off so he could wear them like a big boy. It was mid-afternoon and he refused to take them off and didn't want me to put his nappy back on! I told him if he was going to wear them, then he must try not to wee in them and he must tell Mummy when he needed a wee or poo and I would sit him on the potty. He stayed dry all afternoon until bedtime and we *actually had a battle to get a nappy back on him to go to bed. He finally relented on the promise that I would take it off him again when he woke! The next morning he remembered and wanted the nappy off the moment he woke and still stayed dry in his pants the next day and every day thereafter. Obviously we had the odd accident on occasions but Ollie seems to have a weak bladder that causes him to go to the toilet frequently. Because of this it took us until he was four-and-a-half to get him out of nappies at night. We tried on a few occasions to stop using nappies at night but he would wet the bed two or three times and not even wake – he'd still be sleeping while soaked through! Reducing his drink intake didn't work, and lifting him when we went to bed to get him to do a wee then still meant he wet the bed – he just wasn't ready! I waited until I noticed that his morning nappy was still warm in the mornings and realised he had naturally got to the stage of staying dry overnight and only doing the wee first thing in the morning when he was waking up.*

At age four-and-a-half he was going through a phase where he was very interested in money and getting it as a reward. I therefore decided to offer him a deal. If he brought me his dry nappy in the morning then I would give him 50p. On a Friday when we picked his brother up from school we would go to the shop and he would be able to spend any money he had earned. It worked and he never wet the bed again! Even now at eight years old he still has a very weak bladder. He will go to the toilet every half an hour – an hour during the day and he still gets up 2–3 times every night to go to the toilet!

Ollie was already very used to the potty and toilet for doing a poo. We had terrible constipation problems with him from around six months of age after we began weaning. He had been seen by various doctors, referred to specialists and we had tried lots of medication to get his poo softer and easier to pass, as well as giving him a diet full of fruit and vegetables to help him. Nothing had helped solve the problem completely and we were told by the consultant that it was actually a very common problem and most children grew out of it and began having more regular less painful bowel movements once they were potty trained.

The one thing we had found that helped slightly was sitting him on a potty to do the poo when he began crying and straining. The sitting position meant at least gravity was helping him push it out, rather than him lying on the floor trying to do it in his nappy. Because of this he was very used to a potty already, knew what one was for and was very happy to begin using it to do wees on too.

My daughter was very similar to my firstborn in that she showed all the signs of being ready to begin toilet training around 22 months old. She was telling me before she did a wee and poo, crouching down to do it in her nappy. However, we were travelling abroad on her second birthday for 10 days and I didn't want it to be stressful for me or her while we were on holiday so I delayed starting until we got home. She picked up the idea very quickly with the wee side. The poo side took a few months with her getting the idea to begin with and then regressing slightly after having tonsillitis and a chest infection for a couple of weeks, but at two-and-a-half she had cracked it. She was still in nappies at night, as we planned to do the cot to bed transition first and didn't want too many changes all at once. I never anticipated her being too difficult at night though as her 'daytime nap nappy' was always dry and some mornings her bedtime nappy was too if we got her up as soon as she woke. She easily transitioned to no nappy at night and would call one of us if she needed the toilet in the night or early morning. We had the odd accident, which *was to be expected, but she was dry at night by the time she was three-and-a-half.*

Toilet training comes very easily for some toddlers but needs to be a much slower process for others. They all get there, though, with the usual patience and perseverance. Rushing them, pressuring them and making things stressful will only slow things down and lead to regression, so let your toddler go at her own pace and try not to compare her progress to friends' toddlers or even any previous children you have toilet trained. As with all things where babies, toddlers and children are concerned, lots of patience and perseverance will get you there in the end!

7

Childcare options

Your toddler may already attend a day nursery as part of your childcare arrangements on a daily or weekly basis. If he doesn't, then when he reaches two years old you will need to start thinking about what type of childcare setting you may like him to attend to prepare him fully for starting primary school at four years old. Attending a nursery or pre-school, or using one of the other forms of childcare mentioned, is not obligatory of course. Some parents prefer not to use any form of childcare and care for their child alone or with the help of family or close friends.

Types of childcare

There are three main types of childcare setting to choose from: a day nursery, a Montessori nursery, or a pre-school. Alternatively, for more personalised care, you also have the option of employing a nanny or au pair, or sending your toddler to a childminder.

Day nursery

Day nurseries are generally open for longer hours than a pre-school or Montessori nursery: usually from early morning

(7 or 8am) until early evening (6 or 7pm). They charge a higher daily rate than a pre-school, although some may offer a discount if you have more than one child attending. Day nurseries provide breakfast, lunch and tea as well as snacks and drinks within the price, and most will provide nappies too if needed.

Once your toddler is over three years old, day nurseries will accept the government funding to reduce your monthly nursery bill. Some also accept childcare vouchers that some companies provide to employees as part of their salary. They are inspected by Ofsted (Office for Standards in Education, Children's Services and Skills) to ensure the day nursery provides a safe and stimulating environment for the children in their care.

Pre-school

These are run by qualified staff, as well as some parent helpers, and are generally attached to, or have close links with, a local primary school. Many parents use a pre-school as an opportunity for their toddler to begin mixing with and getting to know some of the children they will be going to school with.

Once your child reaches four years old, the pre-school and feeder primary school will usually arrange taster sessions for them to visit the school before they officially start full time. This helps make the transition to starting school full time a less daunting experience and helps your toddler gain confidence.

Pre-schools generally take children from the age of two or two-and-a-half years and it's worth noting that some prefer children to be toilet trained before starting. This can be a deciding factor for some parents, as day nurseries don't mind if toddlers aren't toilet trained.

The day runs in sessions, usually a 2½–3-hour morning session and the same in the afternoon, and goes along with school-day timings with a 9am start and 3pm finish. Some pre-schools will run a lunch club at an additional cost, but you will need to provide your child with a packed lunch and drink.

The pre-schools that run a lunch club are likely to give you the option of booking your toddler to go for just the morning session, morning plus lunch, lunch plus afternoon, just afternoon or all day 9–3pm.

The government-funding scheme will apply the term after your toddler turns three years old. Pre-schools are inspected regularly and work to the EYFS (Early Years Foundation Stage) curriculum to teach and encourage your child through play activities.

Montessori nursery/pre-school

Montessori nurseries, pre-schools and schools are based on the principles of an Italian doctor called Maria Montessori. The Montessori philosophy relies on having respect for each child as an individual and while the children are guided towards different goals, they are still allowed freedom within their learning environment to select their own way of achieving it. This means that direction and help from adults is kept to a minimum and the aim is that each child effectively teaches themselves.

Not all areas have a Montessori local to them so if this is something you are interested in for your toddler then you may need to travel to find one.

Many Montessori nurseries also group the children in mixed age ranges rather than separating them. The idea is that the younger ones will learn from the older ones and the older ones will help the youngsters.

Theses nurseries are still inspected by Ofsted and usually run in sessions, but a full day can be booked if desired. Vouchers and funding can be used for eligible children.

Childminder

A childminder will care for your child in his own home and should provide a safe and stimulating environment and opportunities for learning and development. Childminders can care for up to six children younger than eight years old, although no more than three of them should be younger than five years old. This number includes their own children if they have any.

Childminders care for a mixed age group of children and their care usually closely mirrors what you would be doing at home from day to day, so many parents feel like it's the next best thing to being at home. Many continue care right up through the school years, if needed, so will do before and after-school drop-off and collection. If you have subsequent children, they can also attend the same childcare setting, meaning you don't need to travel and drop them off in different places.

All childminders have to be registered and inspected by Ofsted so ensure you check those lists when looking at this option. They are trained to follow the EYFS, which is the same structure of learning and care nurseries and pre-schools follow.

When looking for a childminder, ask friends and family who they would recommend locally and then go from there.

Some childminders allow you to use your government funding or childcare vouchers to pay them and they tend to be a cheaper financial option than a nanny or nursery.

Nanny

A nanny is someone you employ to look after your child(ren) in your own home. Most usually have some form of childcare qualification and/or lots of experience and good references from previous families they have worked for. The advantage is that they care for your child in his own home, giving one-to-one care, helping out with the 'nursery duties' such as your children's washing, ironing, cooking, etc., and charge a set weekly fee rather than a per child fee. This makes it a cheaper option if you have more than one child.

You do become an employer, though, and as such have certain obligations to meet. You will have to pay your nanny's national insurance and tax contributions as well as meet certain minimum standards of employment. There are many organisations and nanny agencies that can help you with the technicalities of all this if you would like to explore this option. Nannytax is a company that sorts out the financial side of employing a nanny, providing her with pay slips and letting you know each time a national insurance or tax payment is due. If you employ a nanny who is registered with Ofsted, you may be eligible for help towards your childcare costs each week.

Au pair

Au pairs are usually young people who travel from abroad and are keen to work and study in various countries to improve their English. They usually have little or no childcare training or experience, so it is not a good idea to rely on them to look after children under the age of three years old in a sole charge position. An au pair would live in your house and be useful to help with the care of older school-age children and babysitting, and with the household chores.

Au pairs usually work around 25–30 hours per week in return for receiving their board and lodging and a small amount of money. They usually like to study at the same time at a language centre, or travel. Most au pairs are found though agencies, which match your needs with the details of the au pair. Ensure you use a reputable agency as you will not get to meet the au pair before he or she arrives in the country.

Factors to consider

Your choice of childcare setting will be based on many factors:

Cost

This can be a big deciding factor for many families as the type of childcare you would like and what you can actually afford can be very different. Depending on how many children you have, a change in childcare arrangements may be needed. For example, using a nursery as childcare can work for one child but once you have two or even three children in childcare, then the flexibility of a nanny or au pair may be a better financial option.

Convenience

Are the nurseries/childminders open at the times you need childcare to start and finish so that you and your partner can start and finish work on time? Are they located on your usual journey to work or close to your house to make drop-off and collections easier? Do you have a back-up plan if your child is ill and cannot attend nursery?

The type of learning you want to implement

Nurseries, pre-schools and childminders have to work to a structured guide to provide a stimulating environment for the children in their care and are inspected regularly to ensure they continue to provide that. Do you want to provide that for your child and allow him to interact with his peers or would you rather have one-to-one play and care with a nanny or au pair, and your child enjoying the comfort of his own home?

Your family/working life

Any childcare you choose has to make your life easier and be a positive, not stressful, choice for everyone. Going back to work can be a difficult transition and sending your child to nursery for the first time is a big step (even if you don't have to go to work and will be at home while your toddler attends). It's important to choose childcare that you know will be a welcome addition to your toddler's life in the long term to aid his development, rather than hinder it.

What childcare settings other siblings attend

This is important from a practical point of view. If other siblings are already attending a particular childcare setting or

---

Finding out more

It's always helpful to chat to friends and family members about their own childcare arrangements and what they find works for them. A recommendation from another parent is always a good start when looking for any type of childcare.

Ask around about recommended local nurseries and child-minders and go to visit a few without your toddler to begin with to get a feel for the ones you like. Once you have decided on the type of childcare you would like for your child and have a shortlist, it will be time to involve your toddler in the choice and see how he reacts in the different environments. If you're considering an au pair, invite her round to your home to see how your toddler reacts to her.

school, then any other setting or childcare you choose has to fit in with that and also accommodate older siblings in the school holidays if needed.

Final choice

Once you have decided what type of nursery or pre-school you would like your child to attend, or have decided to use a childminder, then you need to choose which one of the many in your area you would like him to go to.

This decision will now ultimately come down to likeability. I would advise that you book appointments with a selection of nurseries and pre-schools that meet your needs, where the cost, distance and opening hours work for your family circumstances. When you go to the appointment:

- **Take a list of questions.** Ask the same ones at each setting as it will make it easier to compare the answers once you have visited a few.
- **Watch how the staff interact with the children** in their care. Do the children seem happy?

My biggest piece of advice would be to trust your instinct. When you find the right childcare setting for your little one, you will know – it will just feel right. You will be able to imagine dropping off and collecting your toddler and him happily playing there. Even if you have to visit four or five different ones and you don't get that feeling until you visit the sixth, your instinct will let you know when you have found 'the one'.

Settling in

Your final choice of nursery or pre-school should encourage you to bring your toddler in for settling-in days in the lead-up to starting regular sessions on a weekly basis. It's very important to make use of these as they will make for a much smoother transition for your toddler.

The nursery is likely to encourage you to begin the settling-in process by staying with your toddler on the first couple of occasions and then progress to leaving him for a short period of time, so that he understands that you will always return to collect him. You will eventually build up to leaving him to stay for the full session.

These settling-in sessions are very important for both you and your toddler. If this is the first time that he has been left anywhere, or with anyone other than a close friend or family member, it's important that it is a gradual process to avoid any unnecessary upset.

It is very normal for toddlers that haven't ever been away from the family circle to cry on the first few occasions you leave them completely. For most it is the initial separation that is the hardest and as a mum myself and having worked in nurseries, I would advise you keep the goodbye short and sweet. It will be much less painful for both of you and no matter how awful you feel that your toddler is upset, the best thing you can do is stay positive, encourage him to go to his key worker after a kiss and cuddle, and leave.

It's important that your toddler doesn't see you upset, otherwise that will make him think he has something to worry about. Hold it together, wave at the window with a big smile on your face and then once out of sight, you can let go of your emotions and have a good cry!

> **TIP**
>
> *Don't try to sneak away without saying goodbye to your toddler as this will only cause him to be more insecure. No matter how upsetting the farewell may be, it is all part of getting him used to settling in – stay positive and jolly and he will settle down.*

Mummy guilt

Mummy guilt is something that you will already understand and have had experience of many times over now your toddler has reached this age. You will probably feel guilty about anything and everything and how well you are doing as a parent from the moment your little bundle of joy is born. It doesn't seem to be something that affects most fathers – of course they love and care for their children just as much, but in my experience, they seem to be able to switch off to certain things in a way that we as mothers can't.

Mummy guilt will never be something you can stop or control, but you will learn to live with it and knowing that other mums feel the same does help. Think of the Mummy guilt as mother nature's way of making sure we love and care for our children the best we can. You will have reached a point where you know you want your toddler to start pre-school or nursery and are fully aware of the benefits he will get from it, but it won't make you feel any less guilty about sending him, particularly if he cries as you leave him. Call the pre-school or nursery once you get home to see how your toddler is if he was upset as you left. This will reassure you that he has calmed down and is happy despite the sad farewell. Knowing he has settled down and has not been crying all day will hopefully lessen some of the guilt you feel at leaving him.

Once you settle down into regular sessions at nursery, your toddler will become aware of what he is doing on a day-to-day basis – most toddlers will naturally ask this anyway. *My daughter will ask the night before as I'm putting her to bed, 'What are we doing when we wake up, Mummy?' and I will say, 'It's a Mummy day/pre-school day/Ann (her childminder) day.'*

She actually gets more excited on the pre-school days and childminder days than days with me sometimes, unless I have a special treat planned. It's a bit of a kick in the stomach, (yeah thanks for that), but deep down I actually prefer that she's happy to go to other places with confidence and it reassures me and makes my 'Mummy guilt' much less. I know that she enjoys the other places she goes to and won't be upset when I leave her.

Top tips
To help the transition to starting nursery go smoothly:

- **Encourage independent play** some of the time in the lead-up to beginning nursery, so your toddler is not reliant on your presence all of the time.
- **If possible, leave your toddler with close family and friends** for short periods of time before starting nursery. This will help him to gain confidence and independence and be reassured that you will always come back to collect him.
- **Talk about nursery/pre-school in a positive way only**. If your toddler has worries or fears, listen and reassure him. Keep things simple by talking about how much fun he's going to have there. Tell him about the activities he will

do – drawing and dressing up, for example, and playing with lots of new friends.

- **Use your settling-in days.**
- **Build a good relationship with your toddler's key worker,** who you can talk about with your toddler at home.
- **Establish a good home routine and boundaries**, so that your toddler will be used to some structure when he does begin going to childcare.
- **Try to arrive on time** for dropping off and particularly collecting if there are set hours. It is very unsettling for a toddler to try to get involved once activities have already begun in the morning, and much nicer if they can put their coat and bags away at the same time as their peers first thing in the morning. Arriving on time for collection is important for obvious reasons. Nobody wants to be the last child left wondering where Mummy is.
- **Ensure the child carer has details of any comforters** your toddler likes and where they are if needed and also any pet names for special things.

I have worked in various nurseries and pre-schools during my 18-year professional career in childcare and I have also chatted to a few members of staff, who still currently work in them to compile a staff list of helpful things parents can do to make the transition smooth:

- **Dress your toddler in clothes and shoes that don't restrict them** – no flip-flops, for example – and that you don't mind getting dirty or stained. Children need to be able to move freely when climbing and running around. Be aware that the aprons worn during messy play don't always cover all of your child's clothes, so they may get paint on them. Some toddlers will even refuse to wear an apron and so are even more likely to end up with messy clothes – a good rinse in cold water rather than a bio-detergent is the best way to get paint off clothes.

- **Write or put labels on everything** your child brings to pre-school/nursery.
- **Make staff aware of pet names or words for going to the toilet.** One member of staff was slightly stumped when told by a toddler that he wanted to 'rain on Goofy'. It turned out that his potty at home had a picture of Goofy on the base and he was telling her he needed to have a wee!
- **Always provide a change of clothes or even two.** Although childcare providers will have spare clothes, your toddler will feel much more comfortable in his own familiar clothes.
- **Most parents will have to advise of any medical matters** on the registration form, but it's also important to pass on details of any fears or phobias your toddler may have, such as a fear of dogs or spiders or the fact that they are wary of men (a few toddlers, particularly girls, go through a 'scared of men stage').
- **Provide food your toddler likes.** If you provide a packed lunch, then ensure your toddler likes the food. A new setting is not the time to also try to introduce your toddler to new foods.

Twins

Despite being siblings and exactly the same age, twins can be very different. You may have one twin that's more confident and dominant than the other. This may mean that they cope with the idea of starting childcare differently. Treat

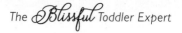

them individually and reassure them if they have any fears or concerns.

If they are starting at the same time, then hopefully the transition will be quite smooth, as having each other there for reassurance will be a big help. It's very likely that the twin that is generally more dominant and confident at home, will continue that at childcare too. As the quieter, more sensitive twin gains confidence, then he will soon settle down and begin to enjoy himself.

Illnesses

If starting childcare is the first time that your toddler has had a chance to mix with other children regularly, then for the first six months at least he will catch quite a few viral infections. Mixing with his peers in a confined space and playing with the same toys will create the perfect environment for viral germs to spread from child to child, no matter how clean and hygienic the equipment and area is kept by staff.

You are likely to find that your toddler catches one cold after another and even gets some of the common infections and diseases that tend to spread easily in childcare environments. Impetigo, hand, foot and mouth disease, chicken pox and conjunctivitis (see Chapter 8) to name a few.

If your toddler is unwell, most nurseries will still charge you the standard daily rate, despite him being unable to attend. Some will try to accommodate you making up the missed day by allowing him to attend on an alternative date, but this will be subject to how busy they are and is not an absolute right you have in most cases. It is totally at the nursery's discretion and not something they have to do. Bear in mind that if you work you will have to take time off to care for your toddler because he's ill and have to use some of your holiday to cater for the time off, until your toddler is able to return to nursery again.

If your toddler is bringing all of these bugs and germs home and getting ill, it's also very likely that you and your partner will catch some of the viruses he gets too. After a few months of coughs, colds and other viruses, you will all build up a stronger immunity and won't get ill as often after that.

If your child attends nursery as part of your childcare arrangements, so that you can go to work, it's worth remembering all of the above.

Funding

All three- and four-year-olds in England are entitled to 15 hours of free early education each week for 38 weeks of the year. Some two-year-olds are also eligible (see below). You can start claiming free early education after your child's third birthday. The date you can claim will depend when your child's birthday falls.

Birthday	When you can claim
1st January–31st March	The beginning of term on or after 1st April
1st April–31st August	The beginning of term on or after 1st September
1st September–31st December	The beginning of term on or after 1st January

Contact your local council for more information about free early education in your area. The free early education can be at:

- Nursery schools
- Nurseries on school sites
- Nursery classes in schools and academies
- Children's centres
- Day nurseries
- Some playgroups and pre-schools
- Childminders
- Sure Start children's centres

Funding for two-year-olds

Some two-year-olds in England can also get free early education. You must be in receipt of one of the following to be eligible:

- Income support
- Income-based Jobseekers Allowance (JSA)
- Income-related Employment and Support Allowance (ESA)
- Support through part 6 of the Immigration and Asylum Act
- The guaranteed element of state pension credit
- Child tax credit (but not working tax credit) and have an annual income not over £16,190
- The working tax credit four-week run-on (the payment you get when you stop qualifying for working tax credit)
- Children looked after by a local council
- The child has a current statement of special educational needs (SEN) or an education, health and care plan
- The child receiving disability living allowance
- They've left care through special guardianship or an adoption or residence order
- You get working tax credits and earn no more than £16,190 per year

If your child is eligible, then you can start claiming free early education after he turns two, depending on when his birthday falls (see table above for cut-off dates, which are the same according to when a two-year-old's birthday falls).

Ofsted

Ofsted is the Office for Standards in Education, Children's Services and Skills. It inspects and regulates services that care for children and young people and those providing education and skills for learners of all ages. It reports directly to parliament and is independent and impartial.

Settings that are inspected by Ofsted include:

- Schools
- Pre-schools
- Nurseries
- Childminders
- Children's centres (children's homes)
- Family centres

Establishments are inspected by Ofsted every three or four years. If the previous inspection went well and the setting was rated good or outstanding, Ofsted may leave it a little longer before the next inspection. If concerns are raised by a parent, there is likely to be an earlier inspection. Ofsted has the power to close childcare settings that do not meet a required standard. There are four gradings:

- Grade 1 (outstanding)
- Grade 2 (good)
- Grade 3 (requires improvement)
- Grade 4 (inadequate)

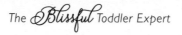

If judged 'requires improvement' or 'inadequate' and has serious weaknesses or requires special measures, the report will explain why. Ofsted will firstly give an establishment time to correct and improve and then will carry out a further inspection to see if the recommendations have been listened to.

Preparing for school

If your child attends a nursery, pre-school or childminder then all of the things they do will help to prepare him for school, from the basics, such as learning to sit down quietly and listen to stories in a group, to encouraging everyone to collectively tidy up and prepare for the next activity.

As your child turns four, most settings will begin to do more structured activities to encourage pencil control, such as following dots and learning to write his own name.

It's crucial that your toddler is encouraged to do this as a fun activity at home too. Practising how to hold a pencil or pen correctly will help him write and follow dots much more easily. Once you find that he can easily follow the dots to write the letters in his name, you could even begin to encourage independent writing.

It is not the nursery's responsibility to teach a child those basic skills, although most will do it as part of their curriculum. How much input and encouragement you give at home to support and develop that learning, will make the vital difference to your toddler's enjoyment and ease at how quickly he takes it all in.

> **TIP**
>
> *Playing picture or word games can help to teach your toddler to recognise numbers 1–10 and the letters and sounds of the alphabet.*

Using any of the above childcare options is a personal choice. It may be an option you need to explore due to work commitments, or you may decide to sign your toddler up for childcare for just a few hours per week to allow you some free time to get things done, even if you don't go out to work. You may, of course, decide you do not want or need to leave your little one with anyone else until he starts school. As long as your toddler is happy, loved and stimulated, then he will thrive in any environment and gradually gain the confidence he needs to prepare him for starting school when the time comes.

8

Common illnesses and problems

During your child's toddler years, she is likely to become ill at times. Most childhood conditions are minor and easily treated. This chapter covers the common ones you are most likely to see or to be aware of, and the symptoms and recommended treatment for each one.

Some of the information included in this chapter has been drawn from the NHS website (see page 309), where you will find an A–Z of illnesses and conditions. This is to ensure the signs, symptoms and treatment advice is as accurate as possible at the time of print. This chapter has also been read by a two qualified GPs who are happy that all of the information provided is correct. As with all concerns regarding your child's health and wellbeing, you should *always* seek the advice of a medical professional if you are at all worried or need reassurance or guidance in addition to the information provided in this chapter.

As a parent it is important that you have a basic knowledge of first aid and you will find many organisations and charities

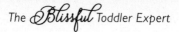

that offer a basic first aid course in your local area for a small charge or donation.

Asthma

In the UK, over 1.1 million children have asthma. It is a common long-term condition that can be effectively controlled, but the severity of the symptoms varies between children, from mild to severe. Asthma cannot be cured, although the majority of children will grow out of it, especially those diagnosed at a young age and those with a mild form of asthma. Asthma is more common in boys than girls when younger, although this changes after puberty when it becomes more common in girls. It can be difficult to diagnose asthma in children as many other conditions can cause similar symptoms.

Asthma affects the bronchial tubes, which carry air in and out of the lungs. In children who have asthma, certain triggers can affect and irritate those tubes, causing them to narrow. The lining becomes inflamed, the muscles around the tubes tighten and there is an increase in the production of sticky mucus or phlegm. This makes it more difficult to breathe and causes symptoms such as:

- Wheezing
- Coughing
- Tightness in the chest
- Shortness of breath

These symptoms can lead to your child having an asthma attack that requires medical treatment.

Causes

Asthma generally runs in families and your child is more likely to have it or develop it if you or your partner have it, or if she was born prematurely or born weighing less than 2 kg (4.5 lb). There is a huge range of 'asthma triggers', although no two asthma sufferers are the same and some can have several triggers. If your child becomes unwell with a cold or flu, it is almost certainly likely to trigger an asthma attack or flare-up of symptoms. Other triggers include:

- Being in an environment where adults smoke
- Exercise, especially in cold weather
- Animal fur
- Pollen
- Grass
- House-dust mites
- Exposure to air pollution, especially cigarette smoke
- Weather conditions and sudden temperature changes
- Food allergies
- Stress

Treatment

While there is no cure for asthma, there are effective treatments to control the condition. Treatment is based on:

- Relieving symptoms
- Preventing future flare-ups

Treatment involves a combination of medicines, usually use of an inhaler to relieve symptoms, a personal asthma action plan and avoiding potential triggers. It is important for your child to continue using prescribed medication with regular reviews. This will help to keep asthma symptoms under control as she gets older. There are several lifestyle changes your GP will discuss with you that will help you manage the condition for your child. With support from the child's nursery and, in time, primary school, there is no reason why a child with asthma cannot take a full part in education and exercise.

Broken bones

If your child has an accident and you think her neck or spine may be injured, call an ambulance immediately. Do not move her as you could cause more damage, and unnecessary movement could cause permanent paralysis. A bone in your child's leg or arm could be broken if she has pain or swelling and it seems to be at a strange angle.

If you are sure the neck and spine are uninjured and have to move your child for safety reasons, be very gentle. Put one hand above the injured limb and one below (or ask someone to help you) to support and steady it. Use blankets or clothing if there is no one around to help. Give infant paracetamol or infant ibuprofen for pain relief and take your child to A&E to get the limb x-rayed and checked.

Burns

Children are very inquisitive and your toddler may not have quite got the hang of what is hot and what is cold to touch. How can she if she doesn't experience touching something hot once or twice?

It is very common for toddlers to experience minor burns from all manner of household items as they explore their surroundings. In general, once they have had an unfortunate encounter with something hot, they do tend to remember it and next time they hear you say the word 'hot' and instruct them not to touch, they are likely to be a little more cautious.

Treatment

- Immediately put the burn or scald under cold running water to reduce the heat on the skin. You can do this for up to 30 minutes if necessary. If there is no running water, then immerse the burned/scalded area in any other cool fluid, such as milk or another cold drink.
- Use something clean and non-fluffy such as a cotton pillow-case, linen tea towel or cling film to cover the burn or scald. This will reduce the danger of infection. If your toddler's clothes are stuck to the skin, don't try to take them off.
- Don't put butter, toothpaste, oil or ointment on a burn or scald as it will have to be cleaned off before treatment by a doctor. Depending on the severity of the burn or scald, see your GP or go to an A&E department.
- Don't burst any blisters that have formed.
- Infant paracetamol and infant ibuprofen can be given for the pain.

Childhood diseases

In the UK, routine vaccinations mean that many childhood diseases – measles, mumps, rubella and whooping cough – that were once very dangerous, are now rare and treatable. However, even if you do vaccinate your child there is still a small possibility that she may contract one of these diseases, although the severity of it will be much less than if she were completely unvaccinated.

Chicken pox

Most children catch this common childhood illness at some point. It is caused by a virus and is spread quickly and easily through the coughs and sneezes of an infected person. It takes 7–21 days for the symptoms to show after you have come into contact with the virus. This is called the 'incubation period'. Someone with chicken pox is most infectious 1–2 days before the rash appears until all of the blisters have crusted over. This usually takes 5–6 days from the start of the rash.

Chicken pox is most common in children under 10 years old and is so common in childhood that 90 per cent of adults are immune to it, as they have had it before. Children usually catch chicken pox in the winter and spring months, particularly between March and May. Due to chicken pox being so contagious, around 90 per cent of people who haven't previously had it will become infected when they come into contact with the virus.

Some children only have a few spots but in others they can cover the entire body. It is possible to get chicken pox more than once, particularly if your child only had a mild case of it and not very many spots. Usually (in most cases) you develop antibodies to the infection first time round and become immune to catching it again. Some people simply don't develop the antibodies needed to protect them against re-infection but experts generally agree that if you have had it once, then you are unlikely to get it again.

Pregnant women are at special risk of serious problems if they catch chicken pox so if your toddler catches it and you haven't already had the virus and are pregnant, seek medical advice as soon as you are exposed to the virus or develop chicken pox symptoms. You can ask for a blood test to check if you are already immune.

Symptoms

- Chicken pox usually starts with a high fever (38°C/100.4°F) for a few days before the rash appears.
- A rash of red, itchy spots that tend to appear in crops and turn into fluid-filled blisters – they then crust over to form scabs, which eventually drop off.
- The spots first appear on the chest, back, head, ears, neck or scalp, then spread to under the arms, the belly, arms and legs – the spots won't leave scars unless badly infected or your child is tempted to pick them. It is very important to discourage scratching or picking to prevent scarring. Distraction and using the treatment options below will help relieve itching and make your toddler less tempted to pick.

Treatment

Chicken pox in children is considered a mild illness and in most cases your child will not need to see a GP. You can expect your child to feel pretty miserable and irritable while she has it and she is likely to have a fever for the first few days. The spots can be very itchy.

To help relieve symptoms for your child:

- Give infant paracetamol for any fever
- Many friends and family members will recommend you dab calamine lotion on the spots to relieve itching, although this is now not recommended medically as when it dries it stops being effective
- Give Piriton as directed by your GP or a pharmacist to relieve itching

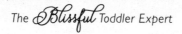

When to see a GP

If the blisters become infected or if your child has a pain in her chest or has difficulty breathing, seek medical advice, as with any other symptoms you are worried about.

Choking

Children, particularly under the age of five years old, often put things in their mouth as a means of exploring. This puts them at a very high risk of choking because if they swallow a small object, it could become lodged in their airway. As parents, it goes without saying that we should all put small objects out of reach to reduce the risk of choking, but accidents happen and young children are very inquisitive, so they may still find something they shouldn't.

If you notice that your child suddenly starts coughing, is not ill and has a habit of putting small things in their mouth, then it is very likely they could be choking. The following information has been taken from the NHS website (see page 309) and is the current advice for a choking child over a year old, at the time of writing:

- If you can see the object, then try to remove it but don't poke around in the mouth if you can't, as you could push something further down.
- If your child is coughing loudly, then encourage her to continue coughing with you there and do nothing else, as any object should dislodge.
- If the coughing is not effective – it's silent or the child can't breathe in properly – shout for help immediately. If the child is conscious but either not coughing at all or the coughing isn't effective, then use back blows as described below.

Back blows for children over one year
- Back blows are more effective if the child is positioned head down.
- Put the child across your lap as you would a baby. If this isn't possible, support the child in a forward-leaning position and give the back blows from behind.

If back blows don't relieve the choking and your child is still conscious, give abdominal thrusts (see below) to children over one year. This will create an artificial cough, increasing pressure in the chest and help to dislodge the object.

Abdominal thrusts for children over one year
- Stand or kneel behind the child. Place your arms under the child's arms and around the upper abdomen.
- Clench your fist and place it between the navel and ribs.
- Grasp this hand with your other hand and pull sharply inwards and upwards.
- Repeat up to five times.
- Make sure you don't apply pressure to the lower ribcage as this may cause damage.

Following chest or abdominal thrusts, reassess your child as follows:
- If the object is still not dislodged and your child is still conscious, continue the sequence of back blows and either chest or abdominal thrusts.
- Call for an ambulance or ask someone nearby to call one for you.
- Don't leave the child.

Even if you get the object out, it is still worth taking your child to an accident and emergency department afterwards, as part of the object may have remained behind or your child may have been injured by your actions.

If the child becomes unconscious, lie her down on a firm, flat surface and call for help. If you can see the object inside your child's mouth, remove it, but if nothing is visible then don't poke around. Wait for an ambulance to arrive.

Conjunctivitis

Conjunctivitis is redness and inflammation of the thin layer of tissue that covers the front of the eye (conjunctiva) and is very common in young children. There are three types – allergic, viral and bacterial conjunctivitis. It can affect one or both eyes. It is highly contagious.

Symptoms
- Itchiness and watering of the eyes
- Red eyes
- Complaining that eyes hurt when they look at lights
- Sometimes a sticky coating on the eyelashes
- A green 'goo' in the corners of the eye that returns very quickly after you wipe it
- Eyes that are stuck together after a period of sleep where the 'goo' has dried and gone crusty

Treatment
In many cases, conjunctivitis doesn't require treatment as symptoms usually clear up within a few days. You can try the following forms of treatment on your toddler to clear up the infection:

- Bathe the infected eye regularly with cooled boiled water. Use one piece of cotton wool once. Wipe from the inside of the eye to the outside and then repeat with a new piece of cotton wool. Use a separate piece for the other eye.
- Wash your hands thoroughly after touching your toddler's eyes as conjunctivitis is very contagious.
- Don't share face cloths or towels while your toddler has the infection.
- Buy an over-the-counter eye cream or drops and begin treating, as per the instructions on the box, once your child is over two years old.

Antibiotics are not usually prescribed for infective conjunctivitis as they rarely make much difference to the recovery. However, if your toddler has a particularly severe case of it or it has lasted more than two weeks, despite you using the above advice and over-the-counter treatment, your GP may prescribe some. It is usually only bacterial conjunctivitis that requires antibiotic treatment (this is usually the one with a yellow/green discharge that keeps appearing in the corner of the eye).

Child carers may insist that your child doesn't attend until the infection is being treated with antibiotics because it is so contagious, but medically there is no need for them to be excluded.

Constipation

This is very common in toddlers once you begin toilet training. The change from doing their poo in a nappy and not really seeing it, to purposefully having to go for a poo on the loo or potty and see the result of a bowel movement, can be scary (see page 170). You may also, without realising it, have created

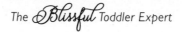

a negative association with poo by jokingly saying from when she was a baby, 'Oh poo, stinky, yucky.' Therefore, by the time you reach the toilet-training stage, your child may be pretty scared by what comes out of her bottom and having to actually see it. This may cause her to hold on to her bowel movement for longer than she should, which if done regularly will make her become constipated.

Being constipated, in turn, makes the poo very painful to pass when the body's natural urge to pass it overrides any reluctance to do. Passing a painful pool can make a toddler even more scared to go to the toilet and so you end up in a vicious circle.

In the toilet training chapter (see page 160), there are stages that I would advise you use to prepare your toddler for toilet training, which will prevent constipation being likely to happen.

If the constipation is diet related or developmental then there are things you can do to help:

- Make sure you aren't giving too much milk. Current daily recommendation of dairy for a toddler is roughly 350 mg of calcium, and around 300 ml (½ pint) of milk will provide this. This allowance is taking into account milk your toddler drinks as well as dairy from the food she eats.
- Make sure your child's diet includes plenty of fibre: fruit and vegetables, baked beans, wholemeal bread or chapattis, wholegrain breakfast cereals, frozen peas and sweetcorn are all good sources of fibre and popular with children.
- Give lots of fluids – ideally water rather than juice.
- Your GP may prescribe a laxative if dietary change doesn't help.

Colds

It is normal for a child to have eight or more colds a year. This is because there are hundreds of different cold viruses and, as they haven't had them before, a young child will have no immunity to them. Each time your child gets a cold she develops an immunity to that particular cold virus and over time, her immunity builds up and she will catch fewer colds.

Starting nursery and mixing with lots of other children means your toddler will pick up far more viral infections to begin with, but it will enable her to build up her immunity more quickly. Most colds get better in 5–7 days. Here are some suggestions on how to ease symptoms:

- Increase fluid intake – encourage your child to drink little and often.
- Give children's ibuprofen and/or children's paracetamol to help ease symptoms, pain and fever.
- Saline nasal drops can loosen dried nasal secretions and relieve a stuffy nose. These can be bought over the counter at a pharmacy.
- Encourage and teach your toddler how to wipe her nose or come and ask you if she needs help. If her nose becomes sore from having to wipe it a lot, you can use a small amount of Vaseline to relieve it.
- Try using a humidifier in your toddler's bedroom at night to help her breathe more easily.
- Encourage the whole family to wash their hands regularly to stop the spread of infection.

Coughs

Children often cough when they have a cold because of mucus trickling down the back of the throat. If your toddler is eating,

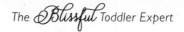

drinking and breathing normally and there is no wheezing, a cough isn't usually anything to worry about. Although it is upsetting to hear your child cough, coughing actually helps clear away phlegm from the chest or mucus from the back of the throat. However, if she has a persistent cough that won't go away, take her to the GP:

- If she also has a temperature over 37.5°C (99.5°F) and is breathless, then she may have a chest infection. If this is caused by bacteria rather than a virus, then your GP will prescribe antibiotics to clear up the infection, although antibiotics won't soothe or stop the cough straight away.
- If a cough continues for a long time, especially if it is worse at night or is brought on by your toddler running about, it could be a sign of asthma (see page 206). Some asthmatic children also have a wheeze or breathlessness. If your child has any of these symptoms, see your GP.
- Once over the age of 12 months, try giving your child a warm drink of honey and lemon to ease the cough.

Croup

Croup is commonly caused by a viral infection and affects the windpipe, the airways to the lungs and the voice box. It usually affects young children aged between six months and three years, with most cases occurring in two-year-olds. About 3 in 100 children will suffer from croup every year. The condition is more common during the late autumn and early winter months, and it tends to affect more boys than girls. It is occasionally possible for a child to experience it more than once during childhood.

Symptoms

Initial symptoms are similar to those of a cold. They include:

- Sore throat
- Runny nose
- Cough
- High temperature (fever) (see page 237)

Over 1–2 days, specific symptoms will develop. These include:

- A bark-like cough
- A hoarse or croaky voice
- Difficulty breathing
- A harsh, grating sound when breathing in, called 'stridor'
- Difficulty swallowing

Symptoms tend to be worse at night, particularly the bark-like cough and stridor. Stridor is often most noticeable when the child cries or coughs. However, in most severe cases of croup it can also occur when the child is resting or sleeping and if this is the case then you need to go to an A&E department as steroid intervention and treatment will be needed. Although symptoms *usually* only last a few days, they can occasionally last up to two weeks in some cases.

Treatment

Treatment depends on the severity of symptoms. Most cases are mild and can be managed at home with:

- Infant ibuprofen to lower a high temperature and reduce swelling (it is more effective than infant paracetamol in this case)

- Plenty of fluids to drink
- Lots of cuddles and TLC to keep your child calm as symptoms often worsen if a child gets agitated or upset

While there is little scientific evidence to support it, some people have found that allowing their child to breathe in steam from a hot bath or shower in a closed room, has eased symptoms. Steam treatment should only be used under careful supervision, as there is a risk of scalding your child. If you use this treatment, ensure you change any clothes your toddler may have been wearing at the time in case they are damp.

If your GP thinks your child has severe croup or symptoms worsen, she may need to be admitted to hospital urgently.

Cuts/scrapes

These are very common because toddlers run around and climb on everything, leading to falls and minor accidents. Grazed knees can be cleaned with cold water to ensure all dirt is removed and ideally then left to heal, with no plaster, as long as they are not bleeding. They inevitably result in a bruise that appears a day or two later and possibly a scab if your child bled at the time of the injury. All of my children as toddlers had shins full of bruises where they took regular tumbles. *You* may think it looks pretty bad, but be reassured that most toddlers' legs are in the same bruised state.

If there is a lot of bleeding coming from a cut, press firmly on the wound with a clean cloth, such as a tea towel or flannel. If you don't have one to hand, use your fingers. Press until the bleeding stops. This may take 10 minutes or more. Don't tie anything around the injury so tightly that it stops circulation.

If possible, raise the injured limb but only if you are not worried it is broken. Raising the limb above the height of the heart will help to stop the bleeding. Cover the wound with a clean dressing. If blood soaks through, then put another dressing on top.

An ambulance isn't usually needed unless there is serious blood loss. However, if the cut continues to bleed, or it looks like it needs to be stitched, then go to A&E to get it checked.

Diarrhoea and vomiting

Some children between the ages of 1–5 pass frequent, smelly, loose stools that may contain recognisable foods such as carrots and peas. Usually, these children are otherwise perfectly healthy and are growing normally, but their GP can't find any cause. This type of diarrhoea is known as toddler diarrhoea. You may find that certain foods trigger certain bowel movements or make your toddler's stools much looser. Make a note of these and avoid giving them if they cause an upset tummy. You can ask your GP to refer your child to a dietary specialist if you think she has an allergy or intolerance to certain foods, in order to confirm a diagnosis. It may mean that long-term dietary changes are needed to help regulate her bowel movements.

You should also contact your GP if:

- Your child has diarrhoea and vomiting at the same time
- Your child has diarrhoea that's particularly watery, has blood in it or lasts longer than two or three days
- It is unusual for your child to have loose stools or her bowel habits suddenly change and you cannot see any reason for it
- Your child has severe or continuous stomach ache

Otherwise, diarrhoea isn't usually a cause for concern.

> ### Tummy ache
>
> *Some toddlers complain of tummy pain when feeling unwell with a virus. This can be due to the glands in their stomach being swollen, from trying to fight off a cold, ear infection, sore throat or other viral infection. Once the infection is dealt with the glands will slowly calm down and the pain should go. In the meantime, a nice warm bath or hot water bottle to hold on the tummy, some pain relief and lots of TLC will help. If you are overly concerned and your toddler seems in a lot of pain, contact your GP for further advice.*

Vomiting

Some toddlers may vomit only once as a reaction to something they have eaten or drunk, or from running around too much, or because they are too hot. There are many different things that can cause vomiting, but if it only happens as a one-off and your toddler seems fine afterwards, then it's usually nothing to worry about. It may have just been her body's way of getting rid of something it didn't like or a slight infection that her antibodies are trying to fight off. You only need to worry if your toddler has repeated episodes of vomiting, i.e. more than twice, and if this happens then it is likely she may have caught a sickness bug.

Treatment

If you think your child does have diarrhoea or vomiting caused by a bug, the following treatment is advised:

- Give your child plenty of clear drinks (such as water or clear broth), to replace the fluid that is being lost. Avoid fruit juice or squash, as these can cause diarrhoea.

- Only give your child food if they want it and try to stick to plain foods to begin with. Avoid dairy products.
- Don't give anti-diarrhoeal drugs as they can be dangerous.
- Oral rehydration prescribed by your GP or bought from your pharmacist can help replace lost fluids.
- Use separate towels and allow your sick toddler her own flannel and towel. Remind everyone else in the house to practise good hygiene and wash their hands after using the toilet and before eating to help stop the spread of infection.
- Don't return your child to childcare until at least 24–48 hours (depending on their policy) after the last episode of diarrhoea or vomiting.
- Don't allow children to swim in swimming pools for two weeks after the last episode of diarrhoea.
- Disinfect all surfaces that an infected person has touched.

Norovirus

Norovirus is the most common stomach bug in the UK. There are at least 25 different strains of noroviruses known to affect humans. They're the most common cause of stomach bugs (gastroenteritis) in the UK. Each year, it's estimated that between 600,000 and one million people in the UK catch norovirus. The illness is sometimes called the 'winter vomiting bug' because it's more common in winter. However, you can catch the virus at any time of the year. The virus is highly contagious and can affect people of all ages and cause vomiting and diarrhoea.

Treatment is the same for any vomiting or diarrhoea bug – give plenty of fluids, encourage rest and gradually re-introduce food to your child when she shows some enthusiasm again. Ensure everyone in household is being very hygienic. Although norovirus can be very unpleasant, it's not usually dangerous and most people make a full recovery within a couple of days without the need to see a doctor. If your child is particularly unwell, do not take her to the GP or hospital before contacting the surgery or hospital by phone first, as you will spread the infection very easily to others.

Ear infections

Ear infections often follow a cold, generally around one week later and sometimes cause a high temperature (see page 237). If your child complains of an earache, either verbally or seems to be pulling or rubbing on one ear, but is otherwise okay, then try giving infant paracetamol or infant ibuprofen for 12–24 hours. Never poke around in your child's ear with cotton buds and only use oil or drops when advised by a GP.

Most ear infections are caused by viruses, which can't be treated with antibiotics and just get better themselves. If symptoms persist, though, take your child back to your GP. After an ear infection your child's hearing may be affected for 2–6 weeks. If a problem seems to last longer than this, then ask your GP for advice. Also, see Glue ear on page 228.

Eczema

Eczema is a long-term condition that causes the skin to become itchy, red, dry and cracked. The most common form is atopic eczema, which mainly affects children but can continue into adulthood. About one in five children in the UK has eczema and mainly develop it before the first birthday. Your child is more likely to get it if there is a family history of eczema.

Atopic eczema usually occurs behind the knees or on the front of the elbows. It is not a serious condition but if your child later becomes infected with the herpes simplex virus, it can cause the eczema to flare up into an outbreak of tiny blisters, called eczema herpeticum and will cause a fever. Two in three children will outgrow atopic eczema by their teens.

Treatment

Although there is no cure for eczema, there are recommended treatments that can help ease symptoms over time. Medications used to treat atopic eczema most commonly include:

- Daily use of emollients for dry skin
- Topical corticosteroids to reduce swelling and redness during flare-ups

Emollients will be prescribed for dry skin and the weakest effective topical corticosteriods. Different strengths are needed for different parts of the body. As long as the eczema is not infected, certain dressing or bandages, known as dry wraps, wet wraps and occlusive dressings, may also be applied by a healthcare professional. They work by reducing itchiness, preventing scratching and helping to stop the skin from drying out. Additional medications will be prescribed as and when needed.

Self-care

As well as using medication, there are things you can do at home to help ease your toddler's symptoms:

- Eczema is often itchy and scratching it can aggravate the skin and eventually cause it to thicken. Scratching the skin also increases the risk of the eczema becoming infected with bacteria. There may be times when your child cannot help scratching, so keep her nails short to minimise the damage. Encouraging her to tap or pinch the skin until the itch has gone may also help.

- Your GP will work with you to establish what might trigger your child's eczema, although it may get better or worse for no apparent reason. If you know there is a particular trigger, you can try to ensure your child avoids it.

- Some foods such as milk, eggs and nuts have been shown to trigger eczema symptoms. However, you should not make any significant changes to your toddler's diet without first consulting your GP, as young children need plenty of calcium, calories and protein that are provided by these foods. If your GP suspects a food allergy, your child may be referred to a dietitian.

- Use emollients to keep your child's skin moisturised and prevent it becoming dry and cracked.

Fits and febrile convulsions

Although fits may look alarming, they're common in children under three years old. Although there are other reasons why children have a fit, a high temperature (see page 237) is the most common trigger. Fever fits, also known as febrile convulsions, become increasingly less common after the age of three and are almost unknown after the age of five. Febrile convulsions aren't usually connected with epilepsy.

The cause of febrile seizures is unknown, although they are linked to the start of a fever – a high temperature of 38°C (100.4°F) or above. There may also be a genetic link to febrile seizures, as the chances of having one is increased if a close family member has a history of them. Around 1 in 4 children affected by febrile seizures has a family history of the condition.

Febrile seizures are quite common. An estimated 1 in 20 children will have at least one febrile seizure at some point. Most febrile seizures occur between the ages of six months and three years, with the average age being 18 months. Although still uncommon, a history of febrile convulsions does lead to an increased risk of epilepsy.

During most seizures the child's body becomes stiff, they may lose consciousness (although not always) and their arms and legs twitch. Some children may wet themselves during the convulsion or immediately afterwards. Although febrile convulsions are common, if your child's temperature goes over 38°C (100.4°F) or 39°C (102.2°F) it doesn't mean you can expect a febrile convulsion. Some children have a high temperature threshold and don't ever experience a febrile convulsion.

My own three children are good examples of this. From babies to this day, if any of them get ill their temperature always soars past 40°C. The highest I have recorded was when my daughter had a bad case of tonsillitis. Her temperature was 42.2°C and yet she still didn't have a febrile convulsion, despite her temperature raging for days.

Treatment

If your child has a fit, she may suddenly turn blue and become rigid with staring eyes. Sometimes the eyes will roll and the limbs will twitch and jerk, or she may suddenly go floppy. The following suggestions will help you deal with the fit:

- Keep calm.
- Lie your child on her side to make sure she doesn't vomit or choke. Don't put anything in her mouth. If you think that she is choking on food or an object, try to remove it.

- Remove your child's clothing and any coverings and make sure she is cool but not chilly.
- Most fits will stop within three minutes. When it is over, reassure your child, make her comfortable and call your GP or out of hours service for advice on what to do next. They may advise you take your child to an A&E department to be checked over or if she seems okay, they may advise you just keep an eye on her.
- If the fit hasn't stopped within three minutes, and you haven't already called for an ambulance, do so now. If it stops but it was your child's first fit, take her to the nearest A&E department to be checked over.
- Try not to panic. Fits need to last longer than 30 minutes for there to be any risk of brain damage.
- Even if it's not the first time and your child recovers quickly, let your GP know that your child had a fit.

Glue ear

Repeated middle ear infections may lead to glue ear, where sticky fluid builds up, and this can affect a child's hearing. It may lead to unclear speech and behavioural problems due to your child being frustrated at not being able to understand and also express herself and her needs effectively. More details on how glue ear can affect language development is explained in a case study on page 134. It is estimated that 1 in 5 children around the age of two years old will be affected by glue ear at any given time and about 8 in every 10 children will have had glue ear at least once by the time they are 10 years old.

Causes

The middle ear is the part of the ear directly behind the eardrum. It is made up of three tiny bones that carry sound vibration from the eardrum to the inner ear. The build-up of fluid associated with glue ear prevents these bones moving freely. This affects hearing because it means the bones can't pass sound vibrations to the inner ear. Exactly what causes this build-up of fluids is unclear, although it seems to be related to a problem with the tube that connects the middle ear to the back of the throat (Eustachian tube). One of the main functions of the tube is to help drain fluid from the middle ear. It's thought that problems with the Eustachian tube may be caused by factors such as a previous ear infection, cigarette smoke inhalation or allergies. Glue ear is not caused by getting water in the ear after swimming and showering or a build-up of ear wax.

Symptoms

The main symptom of glue ear is some hearing loss in one or both ears. This usually feels similar to what you experience when you put your fingers in your ears. Signs that your child may be having hearing problems include:

- Struggling to keep up with conversations as she can't hear properly, or not responding to you when you speak to her
- Becoming aggravated because she is struggling to hear
- Regularly turning up the volume on the TV

Treatment

Most cases of glue ear don't require treatment as the condition will improve by itself, usually within three months. Treatment is normally only recommended when symptoms last longer than three months and hearing loss is significant enough to interfere with speech and language development. In these circumstances, glue ear can usually be treated using minor surgery, which involves placing small tubes (grommets) in the ear to help drain away the fluid.

Hand, foot and mouth disease

HFMD is another viral infection that affects young children. It is highly contagious until a week *after* symptoms begin and is spread quickly in places, such as childcare settings, where there are small groups of children who need to have their nappies changed or who need to use a potty. The infection can spread in the following ways:

- An infected person coughs or sneezes and the contaminated droplets are inhaled or touched on food surfaces, etc.
- An infected person doesn't wash his or her hands properly after going to the toilet and then contaminates surfaces or food (the virus can live for up to four weeks in a person's stools). This makes toddlers who don't wash their hands effectively after a toilet trip particularly good at spreading the infection. Also child carers, who may not practise good hand hygiene.
- Coming into contact with the fluids of an infected person's blisters or saliva.

Symptoms

These usually develop 3–5 days after the initial exposure to the infection. This time is known as the incubation period. Early symptoms include:

- A high temperature, usually around 38–39°C (100.4–102.2°F)
- Loss of appetite

- Cough
- Abdominal pain
- Sore throat
- Occasional vomiting
- Mouth ulcers: after one or two days, red spots develop inside the mouth, particularly around the tongue, gums and inside of the cheeks. At first the sores are the size of a small button roughly. They then develop into larger, yellow-grey mouth ulcers surrounded by a red ring of tissue. You can normally expect to see between 5–10 ulcers in the mouth. They can be very painful and understandably make eating, drinking and swallowing difficult. This can cause a young child to dribble excessively. The ulcers generally pass within 5–7 days.
- Skin rash: soon after the ulcers appear, you will notice small red spots on your child's skin. The most common place for them to develop are on the side of the fingers, back of the hands and side of the heels. They may also develop on the palms of the hands and the sides of the feet, and also the buttocks and groin areas, although these places are less common. The spots are around 2–5 mm in size with a darkish-grey centre and are a 'rugby-ball' type of shape. They are usually painless and not itchy, although occasionally they can progress into small blisters, which can be painful and tender. It is important not to burst any blisters as this can spread the infection. The skin rash and blisters should pass within 3–7 days.

Treatment

Most cases of HFMD will pass within seven days with no medical intervention. If you are unsure whether your child definitely has the disease, you can call your GP or the NHS helpline (see page 309) for advice. You can help ease symptoms for your child by doing the following:

- Offering softer foods so that eating and swallowing is easier and less painful
- Encouraging rest and offering lots of fluids
- Giving infant paracetamol and/or infant ibuprofen to relieve symptoms

Preventing the spread of infection

The best way to avoid catching and spreading HFMD is to avoid close contact with people who have it and practise good hygiene. You should keep your toddler away from any childcare setting while she is feeling unwell. Once she feels better she can return, although some nurseries or schools may refuse admission until the last blister has healed.

Head injuries

When babies first begin to toddle around and try to climb, they can frequently fall over and bang their head. Young children often sustain minor head injuries because they have bundles of energy and no real sense of danger. These common injuries rarely result in any permanent damage.

Symptoms

Minor head injuries often cause a bump or bruise to appear fairly immediately. As long as your child is conscious (awake), with no deep cuts, there is unlikely to be any serious damage. Other symptoms of a minor head injury include:

- A mild headache
- Nausea (feeling sick)
- Mild dizziness
- Mild blurred vision

If your child experiences these mild symptoms after a knock to the head, she won't usually require any specific treatment but you can take her to your GP or A&E department for a check-up if you are worried.

Close observation
After your child has sustained a head injury, observe her closely for 24 hours to monitor whether her symptoms change or get worse.

Signs of a serious head injury
If, following a knock to the head, you notice your child has any of the following symptoms, seek immediate medical attention:

- Unconsciousness, either briefly or for a longer period of time
- Difficulty staying awake or still being sleepy several hours after the injury
- Clear fluid leaking from the nose or ears (this could be cerebrospinal fluid which normally surrounds the brain)
- Bleeding from one or both ears
- Bruising behind one or both ears
- Any sign of skull damage or a penetrating head injury
- Difficulty speaking, such as slurred speech
- Difficulty understanding what people say
- Reading or writing problems
- Balance problems or difficulty walking

- Loss of power or sensation in a part of the body, such as complaining of weakness or loss of feeling in an arm or leg
- General weakness
- Complaining of vision problems, such as significantly blurred or double vision
- Having a seizure or fit
- Memory loss, such as not being able to remember what happened before and after the injury when you ask her to recall the event
- Complaining of a headache
- Vomiting since the injury
- Irritability or unusual behaviour

If any of these symptoms are present, particularly a loss of consciousness (even if only for a short period of time), go immediately to your A&E department or call 999 and ask for an ambulance.

Treatment

If your child has a minor head injury, the advice is:

- Place a cool compress (flannel/kitchen towel with water on) on to the bump or part of the head that sustained the injury
- Give infant paracetamol for a mild headache but avoid NSAIDS (non-steroidal anti-inflammatory drugs) such as infant ibuprofen
- Avoid getting your child too excited – encourage calm, relaxed activities for a few hours afterwards
- Do not have too many visitors
- Make sure you avoid rough play with your toddler for a few days

Take your child to an A&E department if her symptoms worsen or if she develops any new symptoms. If she still has symptoms two weeks after the head injury, or you are unsure about your child returning to nursery or sport then talk to your GP for advice.

Head lice (nits)

This is another one of those taboo subjects. However, it is perfectly normal for children to experience catching nits at least once, particularly if they attend a nursery or pre-school.

The difficulty comes when parents bury their head in the sand, not wanting to believe their child could possibly have head lice and therefore *don't* treat it. This means that those of us who *do* treat our children's hair send them back into pre-school or school, where they are constantly being re-infected. It is one of the most frustrating things I find as a parent.

If your child is showing signs of head lice, treat it as soon as possible. It is not something that will go away. The longer you leave it, the more the head lice multiply, making it a much harder problem to get rid of. It is more likely to need repeated treatments to be eradicated completely.

The facts

Head lice are tiny wingless insects that live in human hair. They are grey-brown in colour, the size of a pinhead when hatched and of a sesame seed when fully grown. They cannot fly, jump or swim and are spread by head-to-head contact, climbing from the hair of an infected person to the hair of someone else. This is why they are a common occurrence in young children as they are more likely to have close contact during play with friends.

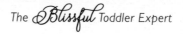

One in three children in the UK will get head lice at some point during the year. Head lice can affect all types of hair, regardless of its condition or length. They are not the result of dirty hair or poor hygiene.

Life cycle of head lice

A female louse lays eggs by cementing them to hairs (often close to the root), where they are kept warm by the scalp. The eggs are pinhead size and very difficult to see in most people's hair (unless you have a major infestation) and have had them a while (see below). After 7–10 days, the baby lice hatch and the empty eggshells remain glued in place. These remains are known as nits. Nits glisten white and become more noticeable as the hair grows and carries them away from the scalp.

Head lice feed by biting the scalp and feeding on blood. They take 6–10 days to become fully grown. Once mature, a head louse can change host and crawl from head to head. A female head louse may start to lay eggs as early as seven days after she has hatched. To break the cycle and stop them spreading, they need to be removed within seven days of hatching.

How to spot head lice

In most cases itching is the main symptom of head lice. It is not caused by the lice biting the scalp but by an allergy to the lice. My boys have had them a few times, particularly my eldest who has longer hair. Most people – adults and children – don't generally scratch their head more than five times per day. When your child has head lice, you will see her scratching a lot, particularly around the back of her head and behind her ears. I always take this as a sign my children have head lice and have a look in their hair.

Not everyone will experience itching and it's not always easy to see head lice, so detection combing is the best way of finding them. This involves using a specialised fine-toothed comb, available from pharmacies. It works better on wet hair and you can comb through for 15 minutes to check the hair or comb for 5 minutes on dry hair.

Even if you can't see or find any lice in the comb, if your child has been actively scratching her head for a few days, it won't do any harm to treat it anyway. Each time I have done this, the itching has stopped, even if I have been unable to find any actual lice, although I have found the nit eggshells.

Treatment

There are various head lice creams and liquids that can be bought over the counter at your local pharmacy. Pregnant women must tell the pharmacist if they are pregnant, so they recommend the correct treatment. If you find that your child has head lice then all household members should be treated. You should then do the detection combing 2–3 days later and then seven days after treatment too.

One thing we have always found is that as soon as the treatment is applied, within five minutes the itching increases to an unbearable amount for about 10–20 minutes. We always joke that it's like the lice are trying to escape the treatment. We usually wait until that mad itching has stopped and then go through with the nit comb and finally wash the treatment shampoo out, and continue to do the detection combing for a week after treatment.

High temperature (fever)

Your child's natural body temperature ranges between 36.5°C (97.7°F) and 37.5°C (99.5°F). A fever is when the body's temperature is significantly higher than normal when the child's temperature is taken by thermometer. A temperature of 38°C (100.4°F) or more in a baby under three months of age and 38.5°C (101.3°F) or more in older infants and children is considered significantly high.

Fever is the body's natural response to help fight infections. It increases the body's normal temperature, which in turn stimulates the immune system (the body's natural defence against infections and illness). A fever makes it more difficult for the bacteria and viruses that cause infections to survive. A fever itself is not harmful, so it is usually not necessary to treat it. However, children with a fever often feel uncomfortable and unwell, so giving pain relief medication such as infant paracetamol and/or infant ibuprofen may be helpful to ease any discomfort.

A fever that does not respond to infant paracetamol or infant ibuprofen is no worse than a fever that does. A high fever does not always mean your child has a serious illness. If your child's fever becomes too high, though, she may end up having a febrile convulsion (see page 226).

Treatment
- Lots of fluids
- Don't sponge your child with water or use a fan to cool her down – she may feel cold even though she has a high temperature
- Dress your child in enough clothing so that she is not shivering or sweating and is comfortable
- Give infant paracetamol and/or infant ibuprofen as directed if she feels unwell
- Watch for signs that she may be getting worse – other symptoms such as vomiting, complaining of aches and

Thermometers

- **Ear thermometers:** These use an infrared ray to measure the temperature inside the ear canal. They are not uncomfortable to the child and generally give a very fast reading. However, you have to ensure you insert it as per the instructions to get an accurate reading. I usually take the reading three times with my own children to make sure I get roughly the same result each time and am reassured it's accurate. This type of thermometer is only recommended for babies and children over six months.

- **Oral thermometors:** Only recommended for children over four years old who can safely hold it in their mouth, under their tongue, for the recommended amount of time.

- **Temporal artery thermometers:** These are the newest and most expensive type of thermometer and used in many hospitals. They use an infrared scanner to measure the temperature of the temporal artery in the forehead. They are safe, fast and not intrusive to use at all. These are different to the basic and very cheap, strip-type thermometers, which aren't very accurate as they show the skin temperature and not the body temperature.

- **Under arm (axillary) thermometers:** These are the cheapest type of thermometer but will still be accurate if you follow the instructions. You have to hold the thermometer under your child's arm until the beeper sounds to tell you the reading. It does mean you have to hold your child still for around 20 seconds, but a cuddle while sitting on your lap and taking the temperature at the same time, will give you an accurate reading.

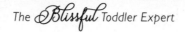

pains or becoming difficult to rouse and keep awake for any length of time.

- Consult a GP if there no improvement or she gets sicker

Most viruses cause a fever with cold symptoms but not all. If you feel that your child needs to see a GP at any point, don't hesitate to take her. If she still doesn't improve a couple of days later, and you are worried, then take her back. As parents we all have to trust our instincts – we know our children best. If you feel that something is wrong, then be insistent and get a second opinion. Most GP surgeries will not question seeing an unwell child repeatedly if the parent is worried and will be happy to listen and reassure you.

Impetigo

Impetigo is a highly contagious skin infection that causes sores and blisters. It's very common in young children because their immune system has not fully developed, making them more vulnerable to such infections.

Infection can occur when bacteria invades otherwise healthy skin through a cut, insect bite or other injury. This is known as *primary impetigo*. An infection can also occur when the bacteria invades the skin as a result of the skin barrier being disrupted by another underlying skin condition, such as head lice (see page 235), scabies or eczema (see page 224). This is known as *secondary impetigo*.

An impetigo infection can spread to other people through physical contact or by sharing towels or flannels. As the condition doesn't cause any symptoms until 4–10 days after initial exposure to the bacteria, it is often easily spread to others unintentionally. There are two types:

- Bullous impetigo causes large painless, fluid-filled blisters
- Non-bullous impetigo, which is more contagious, causes sores that quickly rupture (burst) to leave a yellow-brown crust

Treatment

Impetigo usually gets better on its own within 2–3 weeks. However, it is advisable to see your GP, who is likely to prescribe an antibiotic to prevent the spread of infection, particularly to other family members. If your child attends school or nursery, she is unlikely to be able to return until antibiotic cream is prescribed. A child is unlikely to be contagious 48 hours after treatment, once the sores have dried and healed. To minimise the risk of the infection spreading:

- Avoid touching the sores
- Wash your hands and your toddler's hands regularly
- Don't share flannels, bed sheets or towels
- Keep your child off nursery/school until the sores have dried up

Ingesting a poisonous substance

Young children are very curious and to begin with do not understand the dangers that many household products, substances and medicines pose. It is important that you keep anything that poses a safety risk to your child stored safely away in a locked cupboard or in a place she cannot reach easily. If, despite the safety measures you have taken, you think your child has swallowed pills or medicines, follow the guidelines below:

- Unless you're absolutely sure, spend a minute or two looking for the missing pills (have they rolled under a chair? It's very easy to panic at times like this.)

- If you still think your child has swallowed something, take her to your GP or A&E department, whichever is quickest.
- Take the full set of tablets with you, so that medical professionals can check the labelling and calculate how much your child may have taken. If you don't have the packaging for the medication, write down what you think your child may have swallowed.
- Don't give salt and water, which was advice that used to be given years ago and may still be given by a well-meaning relative or friend, or do anything else to try to make your child sick.

If you think your child has swallowed household/garden chemicals:

- Stay calm yourself so that you can keep your toddler calm. Act quickly to get her to hospital.
- If possible, write down the name of whatever you think she has swallowed or take the packaging.
- If your child is in pain or there's any staining, soreness or blistering around her mouth, she has probably swallowed something corrosive. Give her milk or water to sip in order to ease the burning and get her to hospital quickly.

Measles

Measles is a highly infectious viral illness. It is very rare now in the UK due to the effectiveness of the MMR vaccination. Anyone can get it if they haven't been vaccinated or had it before, but it's more common in children aged between 1–4 years old. The measles virus is contained in the millions of tiny droplets that come out of the nose and mouth when an infected person coughs or sneezes. It spreads easily and is caught by breathing in these droplets, or by touching a surface that has been contaminated with these droplets and then touching your own nose or mouth.

The most effective way of preventing measles is the measles, mumps and rubella (MMR) vaccine. The first MMR vaccine is given at around 13 months old and a booster is given before a child starts school. If your child is younger than 13 months and you think she may have been exposed to the measles virus, see your GP immediately. The MMR may be given if a child is over six months or she may be given antibodies for immediate protection if she is younger than six months.

Symptoms

Initial symptoms include:

- A mild-severe temperature, which may peak at over 40.6°C (105°F) for several days, then fall but go up again when the rash appears
- Red eyes and sensitivity to light
- Tiredness, irritability and general lack of energy
- Aches and pains
- Poor appetite
- Dry cough
- Greyish/white spots in the mouth and throat
- After 2–4 days, a red-brown spotty rash appears. It usually starts behind the ears and spreads around the head and neck before spreading to the legs and the rest of the body. The rash can last for up to eight days.

Treatment

There is no specific treatment for measles as it is a viral illness. The immune system should fight off the infection within a couple of weeks. In severe cases, hospital treatment is needed. Although vaccinated children are unlikely to catch it, you should keep a child with measles away from other children for at least five days after the rash has appeared. There are several things you can do to help your child feel more comfortable:

- Close the curtains to help reduce light sensitivity
- Use damp cotton wool to clean the eyes
- Give infant paracetamol or infant ibuprofen to relieve fever, aches and pains
- Offer plenty of water to drink to prevent dehydration

Meningitis

This is one of the most frightening infections that your child has a risk of developing, mainly because the symptoms are so similar to a general virus and therefore difficult to stop. As a mother of three children myself, this infection is the one I have always feared the most.

Meningitis is an infection of the meninges (protective membranes) that surround the brain and spinal cord. The infection causes the meninges to become inflamed, which in some cases can damage the nerves and brain.

Children in the UK now receive a vaccination for meningitis C as part of their childhood vaccination programme. The meningitis C vaccine does not protect against meningitis caused by the group B bacteria, so it is important to still be aware of the symptoms. The vaccination for the meningitis B strain will be rolled out into the UK national vaccine programme very soon, although it is already available if you would like to pay for it privately. Ask your GP to arrange this. There are two types of meningitis:

- Bacterial meningitis is caused by bacteria and can be spread through close contact, such as kissing, where saliva and mucus are exchanged. This is very serious and should be treated as a medical emergency. If the infection is left untreated it can cause severe brain damage and infect the blood (septicaemia). It is most common in children under five years old and, in particular, babies under the age of one. It is also common among teenagers aged 15–19.
- Viral meningitis is the most common and less serious type of meningitis. Symptoms are often so mild they are mistaken for flu. It is most common in children and more widespread during the summer months.

Signs and symptoms in children for viral meningitis
- Very high temperature (above 37.5°C/99.5°F) but the hands and feet feel cold
- Acting agitated and not wanting to be touched
- Some children can become *very* sleepy and be difficult to rouse
- May appear confused and unresponsive
- Complaining of a stiff neck and the light hurting their eyes
- Not passing urine
- Fast breathing
- Complaining of a headache or pains in the head
- May cry continuously
- They may develop a blotchy red rash that does not fade when you roll a glass over it (although not all children will get this rash). The rash is generally the last symptom to appear and can indicate the infection is now very serious. Don't wait for the purple rash to appear as not every child will get it. It is very important that you seek medical help if you notice any of the above symptoms in your toddler, even if it is the middle of the night.

Treatment

Viral meningitis usually gets better within a couple of weeks with bed-rest and painkillers.

When bacterial meningitis is suspected, treatment will usually start before a full diagnosis is confirmed, as it is dangerous to delay treatment while waiting for test results to come back.

Bacterial meningitis is treated with antibiotics intravenously, directly through a vein in the arm. Treatment requires hospital admission and if severe your child will be admitted to the ICU (Intensive Care Unit). At the same time your child may also be given:

- Oxygen
- Steroids to help reduce the swelling around the brain
- Fluids intravenously

Molluscum contagiosum (MC)

MC is a viral infection that affects the skin. It is highly contagious and very easily spread. It is caused by the molluscum contagiosum virus (MCV). Most people have developed a natural immunity to the MC virus, which means that they will not develop it even if they come into contact with it. However, some people with weak a immune system, such as young children and those with health conditions, are most at risk. If your child becomes infected and spots appear on her skin, the infection is likely to spread among toddlers in a childcare setting, while playing and sharing toys. It isn't known how long someone remains contagious for, but it is thought up until the last spot has completely healed. MC can be spread through:

- Close direct contact – touching the skin of an infected person
- Touching contaminated objects, such as towels, flannels, toys and clothes

Symptoms

Usually the only symptom of MC is a number of small, firm raised spots that develop on the skin. They are not painful, but may be itchy. Generally one or two may appear and then a few more all in the same area to begin with. Visit your GP if you suspect your child has MC.

Treatment

Unfortunately, there is no treatment for most cases of MC. You generally have to wait for the virus to run its course, which can take 12–18 months in some cases. In children who have a weakened immune system because of other health issues, then MC can last much longer. A number of various topical creams, lotions and ointments can be prescribed, which will relieve symptoms.

For most cases of MC in children, the virus doesn't cause any other symptoms apart from the spots and it doesn't interfere with daily activities, so it's best to allow it to clear up over time. Although MC is highly infectious, most people are resistant to the virus and unlikely to develop it, even if they come into close contact with it.

We had one child have a particularly bad case of MC at a nursery I worked in and none of the other children got infected at all. A child I was a nanny to also had a bad case of it on her hands when my son was younger. They had close contact for months and it never spread from her to my son. It is therefore not necessary to keep your child away from nursery or to stop doing activities such as swimming.

Treatment is usually only recommended for older children and adults in cases where the spots are particularly unsightly and affect quality of life. MC doesn't usually cause complications but in rare cases the spots can become infected with bacteria. This is more likely to happen if your child has atopic eczema (skin irritation caused by allergy), or if your toddler has a weakened immune system.

If the spots do become infected, your child will need antibiotic treatment. *Do not* squeeze the spots because it can cause pain, bleeding and an increased risk of spreading the infection and is also likely to cause scarring. You can take steps to avoid spreading the virus to people who are less resistant:

- Keep affected areas of skin covered with clothing, where possible
- Avoid sharing towels, flannels and clothing
- Avoid sharing baths
- Discourage your child from scratching as it can encourage the infection to spread to other areas and take longer to clear up

Mumps

Mumps is a contagious viral infection that used to be common in children. Before the introduction of the MMR vaccine in 1988, mumps was a very common infection in school-age children. It was responsible for about 1,200 hospital admissions a year in England and Wales. It is much less common now with the majority of cases occurring in people born between 1980–1990 who didn't receive the MMR vaccine as part of their childhood vaccination schedule, or who had the mumps virus as a child.

Symptoms

The symptoms of mumps usually develop 14–25 days after a person is infected with the mumps virus. The average incubation period is around 17 days. The symptoms are:

- Swelling of the glands at the side of the face under the ears, giving a person with mumps a distinct 'hamster face' appearance. Both glands are usually affected, although sometimes only one gland is affected. The swelling can cause pain, tenderness and difficulty with swallowing.
- Headache
- Joint pain
- Feeling sick
- Dry mouth
- Mild abdominal pain
- Feeling tired
- Loss of appetite
- A high temperature of 38°C (100.4°F) or above
- Pain and swelling in one, or sometimes both testicles

Treatment

There are currently no anti-viral medications that can be used to treat mumps. Treatment is focused on relieving symptoms until the body's immune system manages to fight off the infection. If symptoms don't improve after seven days or worsen then take your child to the GP.

The following should help:

- Bed rest until symptoms have passed
- Infant ibuprofen or infant paracetamol to relieve pain

- Drinking plenty of fluids, although avoid giving acidic drinks such as fruit juice, as these can irritate the facial gland (see above) – water is best
- A warm or cool compress on the swollen glands to help reduce pain
- Foods that don't require a lot of chewing, such as soup, mashed potatoes and scrambled eggs

If your child has mumps, it's important to prevent the spread to others. The best ways to do this are:

- Keep your child off school or nursery for five days from the onset of the swollen glands
- Wash her hands regularly using soap and water
- Always encourage your toddler to use a tissue to cover her mouth and nose when she sneezes or coughs and then throw the tissue in the bin straight away

Objects put in the nose or ears

Children put things in all sorts of places, even up their own nose and in their ears. One of my earliest childhood memories is putting a pea up my own nose. Our neighbour held one nostril closed and told me to blow it out as if I was blowing my nose on a tissue and hey presto, out it flew, much to the relief of my mother who had completely gone into panic mode!

If your toddler has something up her nose or in her ear, don't try to remove it manually as you may push it further in. If her nose is blocked, show her how to breathe through her mouth and take her to your nearest A&E department.

Pre-school booster vaccination

As part of the UK vaccination programme, your child will have the second dose of the MMR vaccine (what is commonly known as the 'pre-school booster') after she turns three years old. You will receive a letter from your GP surgery at this time. This 4-in-1 booster vaccine is given to three-year-old children to boost their protection against:

- Diphtheria
- Tetanus
- Whooping cough
- Polio

Children are routinely offered these vaccinations as babies in the UK and this booster increases their immunity even further.

How effective is it?

In clinical trials, more than 99 per cent of children who had been given the pre-school booster developed protection against tetanus, diphtheria, whooping cough and polio. The vaccines protect children from these infections until they receive their teenage booster between the ages of 13–18.

Side-effects of the vaccination

Not all children will have side-effects after the vaccination, but if they do these are most likely to happen within 48 hours of the injection being given and include the following:

- Loss of appetite
- Mild fever
- Restlessness

- Irritability
- Crying
- Pain, redness and swelling at the injection site

Keep an eye on your child after the vaccination, give infant paracetamol and/or infant ibuprofen if needed and contact your GP if you are worried about any adverse or unusual side-effects.

Rashes

Childhood rashes are very common and often nothing to worry about. Most rashes are harmless and go away on their own.

Causes

Some things that can cause rashes:

- Heat – being too hot
- Allergic reaction to creams, washing detergent, new clothing, etc
- Pets
- Cold viruses

In most cases a rash will go within 24–48 hours and your toddler will show no other symptoms. However, if your child has developed a rash and seems unwell, or if you are worried that it looks unusual or covers a large part of her body then you should always see your GP as a precaution and for reassurance to rule out anything more serious or a contagious infection.

Rubella

Rubella (also known as German measles) is a mild viral infection that used to be common in children before the introduction of the MMR vaccine. It is spread in the same way as other viral infections, by inhaling a rubella-infected droplet of moisture from someone who is infected. These droplets are released into the air when someone coughs, sneezes or talks.

Symptoms

The symptoms take 2–3 weeks to develop after someone is infected with the rubella virus. During the incubation period, some people may have a slightly raised temperature, conjunctivitis or feel like they are getting a cold. After the incubation period the main symptoms are:

- A distinctive red-pink spotty rash, which may be itchy. It usually starts behind the ears, before spreading around the head and neck. It may then spread to the trunk (abdomen and chest), legs and arms. The rash usually lasts 3–7 days.
- Swollen lymph nodes (glands). Swelling usually appears behind the ears, below the skull at the back of the head and in the neck. This can be very painful and sometimes the glands can be swollen before the rash appears and can last for a week after it has disappeared.
- A high temperature – a fever of 38°C (100.4°F), which can remain high for several days.
- Cold-like symptoms, such as a runny nose, watery eyes, sore throat and cough.

Treatment

There is no specific treatment for the rubella infection. The condition is usually mild and improves without treatment and symptoms disappear within 7–10 days. Do not take your child to the GP unless advised to do so (due to spreading the infection). The rash itself does not need any treatment. It usually disappears within a week. You should:

- Keep your child from childcare settings for four days from the start of their rash
- Keep her away from any pregnant women for at least one week after the start of the rash, unless you know the mother-to-be has been vaccinated against rubella

To relieve other symptoms:

- Give infant paracetamol or infant ibuprofen to reduce fever and treat any aches and pains
- Offer plenty of fluids
- Use a cool (but not cold) compress, such as a damp flannel, to reduce a high temperature
- Cough medicines will be of little help. The best treatment is to put a bowl of water in the room, which will increase the humidity and help relieve the cough. If the radiators are on, you can put a wet towel on them, which will release more water into the air. Warm liquids to drink may help relax the airway, loosen mucus and soothe a cough.

Slapped cheek syndrome (SCS)

This viral infection, also known as 'fifth disease', most commonly affects children between 6–10 years old. However, if your child attends nursery or another childcare setting, she is more likely to come into contact with it from peers who have caught it from older siblings.

Symptoms

Initial symptoms are flu-like but because they are similar to a general cold or virus often no action is taken. This is the point at which your child is most contagious (and why this infection spreads in schools and nurseries). There is a period of 7–10 days with no symptoms, which is then followed by a rash that progresses in three stages:

- **First stage:** 75 per cent of children will develop a bright red rash on both cheeks (the so-called 'slapped cheeks'). It is particularly noticeable in bright sunlight and usually fades after 2–4 days.
- **Second stage:** 1–4 days after the appearance of the 'slapped cheek' rash, a light pink rash usually appears on your child's chest, stomach, arms and thighs. This rash often has a raised, lace-like appearance and may be itchy. By this time your child is no longer contagious and can return to her childcare setting. The rash will fade and go after a few days.
- **Third stage:** In some cases the rash can continue to fade, then re-appear for weeks after the infection has passed. This can be triggered by exercise or if your child becomes hot, anxious or stressed.

Treatment

There is no vaccination for SCS. It is usually a mild illness and will clear up without any medical treatment. You can make your toddler more comfortable and relieve symptoms by offering:

- Infant paracetamol and/or infant ibuprofen to bring down a high temperature (see page 237) or relieve pain
- Antihistamines to relieve itchy skin

- Moisturising lotion on itchy skin
- Rest and fluids as this will help with sore throat symptoms and a high temperature
- You should keep your toddler away from any friend or relative who may be pregnant and if you yourself are pregnant, seek medical advice. There can be severe complications and even death to the unborn baby if the mother catches it.

Sore throat

Sore throats are often caused by viral illnesses, such as a cold or flu. Your child's throat may be dry and sore for a day or two before a cold starts. Infant paracetamol and/or infant ibuprofen can be given to reduce the discomfort. Most sore throats clear up on their own after a few days. If your toddler has a sore throat for more than three days, has a high temperature (see page 237) and is generally unwell or is unable to swallow fluids, then see your GP. Your child may have tonsillitis, which will need treating with antibiotics.

Tonsillitis – inflammation of the tonsils

The tonsils are two small glands that sit on either side of the throat (if you look inside your toddler's mouth and ask her to say 'ahhh', you should see them at the back). In young children the tonsils help to fight germs and act as a barrier against infection. When the tonsils become infected, they isolate the infection and stop it spreading further into the body. As a child's immune system develops and gets stronger, the tonsils become less important and usually shrink. In most people the body is able to fight infection without the tonsils.

Causes

Tonsillitis is usually caused by a viral infection – some cases can also be caused by a bacterial infection. There are a few main signs that tonsillitis is caused by a bacterial infection rather than a viral infection and may need treatment with antibiotics:

- A high temperature (see page 237) that has lasted more than four days
- Being unable to eat or drink due to the pain it causes
- White pus-filled spots on the tonsils
- Swollen and tender lymph nodes

Treatment

- Infant paracetamol and/or infant ibuprofen medicine to relieve pain and reduce a high temperature
- Drinking plenty of fluids
- Rest

If your child has bacterial tonsillitis, a short course of oral antibiotics may be prescribed, which usually relieves symptoms within 24–48 hours. In most cases, tonsillitis gets better within a week. However, a small number of children and adults have recurrent tonsillitis, and surgery to remove the tonsils may be needed. Because the tonsils' job is to stop infection going down into the body, surgery is only recommended in cases where there have been several episodes over a long period of time, as in most cases it is better to leave the tonsils in to stop infection going further than the throat.

My eldest son had to have his tonsils removed when he was four years old after repeated monthly bouts of bacterial tonsillitis. He would be very poorly for a week each time and it would take a

10-day course of antibiotics to fight the infection every time. After 18 solid months of repeated infections from the age of 2–4 years old, he had a tonsillectomy (tonsils removed). For us and him it was the best decision possible, because of all the repeated infections and him having to take antibiotics for one week in every month. In the eight years since then I can honestly count on one hand the times he has been unwell, so that reassures us that the right decision was made for our circumstances.

Splinters

With all the climbing and exploring children love to do, it is inevitable that at some point they will get a splinter under the skin on their finger. There are not many toddlers who will sit still long enough for you to remove a splinter with tweezers but, by all means, try that method first if the splinter looks easy to remove. Ensure you sterilise the tweezers first using an antibacterial wipe or by placing them in boiling hot water for a few minutes. The baking soda (bicarbonate of soda) method is used by many parents and is an easy, fairly pain-free way to remove a splinter:

1. Make a thick baking soda paste by adding water to about a quarter of a teaspoon of baking soda.
2. Wash your hands and then clean and dry gently the affected area with soap and water.
3. Apply the paste to the splinter: spread it on to a bandage, then apply the bandage to the affected area. The baking soda paste will cause the skin to swell and push the splinter out.
4. Leave the bandage on overnight. The splinter may be sticking out of the skin. If it's visible, pull it out with tweezers and rinse the skin.

5. If it still seems embedded, then repeat the steps above for another 24 hours. If the skin seems swollen, inflamed or infected around the splinter, it is advisable to seek medical advice.

Styes

A stye is a small abscess (painful collection of pus) on the eyelid. It appears as a painful lump on the outside or inside of the eyelid. It is fairly common for people to have one or two styes during their lifetime.

Causes

A stye is usually caused by an infection with *Staphylococcus* bacteria, which often live on the skin without causing any harm. It can also be caused by one of the following:

- An infection of an eyelash follicle (a small hole in your skin that an individual eyelash grows out of).
- An infection of the sebaceous gland – this gland is attached to the eyelash follicle and produces an oily substance called sebum, which lubricates the eyelash to prevent it drying out.
- An infection of the sweat gland that empties into the eyelash follicle; the fluid joins the tear film that covers the eye and prevents the eye from drying out.

Symptoms

Symptoms include:
- A watery eye
- A red eye or eyelid

Treatment

A stye often gets better without any treatment, particularly after it bursts and has released pus. Most styes should go away within 1–3 weeks. *Do not* try to burst the stye yourself. The treatment below will ease symptoms:

- Use a warm compress – a cloth or flannel warmed with hot water. Be careful not to make it too hot. Hold the warm compress over the affected eye for 5–10 minutes. Repeat this 3–4 times a day until the stye either clears up or releases some pus.
- The warmth of the compress encourages the stye to release any pus, which will drain away. After this, symptoms should quickly improve. Keep the area around the eye clean and free from crusting. Painkillers such as infant paracetamol and/or infant ibuprofen can be given if you think your child is in pain from the stye.

My daughter had a stye when she was aged two-and-a-half. She had been perfectly fine going to bed and then when I got her up, I noticed a lump on her lower eyelid. I knew what it was and after looking on the NHS website and speaking to a pharmacist, the treatment of a warm compress was recommended. I was told I didn't need to see our GP and to persevere with the warm compress. I used the compress 4–5 times per day, but unfortunately not as long as the recommended 5–10 minutes each time. Trying to get a toddler to sit still and allow me to hold a flannel on her eye for that long just wasn't happening!

We turned it into a bit of a game and would count to 10 as I held it on her eye. We would manage three lots of 10 before she would become bored and want to stop. We continued this treatment for four days and noticed the stye improving and going down in size slowly each day. It didn't ever burst or produce any pus, but gradually disappeared by day seven without us having to visit the GP.

Threadworms

Threadworms, also known as pinworms, are tiny parasitic worms that hatch eggs in and infect the large intestine. They are the most common type of worm infection in the UK, particularly in children aged under 10.

This is unfortunately one of those lovely childhood conditions that no parent wants to encounter or talk about. However, if your child attends childcare and is a thumb- or finger-sucker, it is highly likely you will experience these at some point. Even if you teach your child to practise good hygiene skills, she is still at risk of catching worms from basic contact with other infected children.

Symptoms

Threadworms often go unnoticed by people who have them but symptoms include:

- Intense itching around the anus (or vagina in girls) particularly at night when the female worms come out of the bottom briefly to lay more eggs
- Disturbed sleep as a result of itching, which can lead to irritability
- You may spot threadworms on bedclothes or sheets at night, or notice them in your child's stools. They look like threads of white cotton about ½ in (1 cm) long. It's worth having a quick look at your toddler's poo before flushing it away.

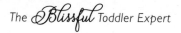

A white wriggly threadworm is easy to spot in a poo and I am speaking from experience with my own child.

It's important to be aware of the symptoms and treat threadworms. Left untreated, the condition will persist and become more severe. It can then cause:

- Loss of appetite
- Weight loss
- Bedwetting
- Difficulty getting to sleep or staying asleep
- Skin infection around the anus

My eldest son is a thumb-sucker, so after working in nurseries for years, I knew he was at high risk of catching worms at some point. The first time he contracted worms he was three years old. He was pretty poorly at the time with tonsillitis and it was around 10pm when he woke crying to have a top-up of medicine. He went to the toilet and then jumped into bed afterwards but was very wriggly, so I asked him what was wrong. He said, 'Mummy my bum tickles.' Knowing what I know after working in childcare for so long, I checked his bottom to see if my fears were correct. Sure enough there was a little white threadworm that wriggled out of his bottom as I looked, and disappeared back in just as quickly.

I was mortified, but of course couldn't tell him what I had seen late at night, for fear of terrifying the poor child. The next day we went to the GP who prescribed treatment for the whole family. The recommendation is always to treat the whole family as a precaution, even if no one else shows symptoms. Usually a visit to the GP is not needed as treatment can be bought over the counter for the whole family, but as it was the first time I had actually seen a threadworm I wanted to speak to my GP first. My eldest son has since had it twice more and none of the rest of us have caught it, but we have still taken the medication as a precaution and just bought it over the counter at the pharmacy, without needing to see the GP again Now he checks his own poo before flushing it away, although the thumb-sucking at school stopped a while ago, so thankfully we have had no more occurrences.

Treatment

To successfully treat threadworms, all household members must be treated, even if they are showing no symptoms. This is because the risk of infection spreading is very high. The aim is to get rid of the threadworms and prevent re-infection. This involves a combination of medication to kill the worms and strict hygiene measures to stop the spread of the eggs. The main medication used to treat threadworms is available to buy over the counter at your local pharmacy, without prescription. You only usually need to see a GP if any family member who needs treatment is under two years or you are pregnant or breastfeeding. Your GP may prescribe an alternative treatment in those instances.

The medication is 90–100 per cent effective at killing the threadworms, but it doesn't kill the eggs. The hygiene measures below should be followed for six weeks as the lifespan of a threadworm is approximately that long:

- Wash all nightclothes, bed linen, towels and soft toys at first diagnosis. It is fine to use the normal washing machine temperature.
- Hoover and dust the whole house regularly, paying particular attention to bedrooms.

- Clean the bathroom and kitchen regularly.
- Avoid shaking any material that may be contaminated with eggs, such as clothing and bed sheets – this helps stop eggs being transferred to other surfaces.
- Don't eat food in the bedroom because you may end up swallowing eggs that have been shaken off on the bedclothes.
- Keep fingernails short – eggs end up under the nails after night-time itching and are then transferred on to food and household surfaces to infect other people.
- Discourage nail-biting and finger- and thumb-sucking as this increases the risk of worms, although as a mother of two thumb-suckers, I know this is a very hard task.
- Wash hands frequently and scrub under the nails before eating, after going to toilet and after changing nappies.
- Give your child close-fitting underwear at night and change it every morning, even if they don't usually wear underwear. It's good to encourage use while treating the threadworm infection.
- Bath or shower regularly, particularly first thing in the morning.
- Don't share towels or flannels.
- Keep toothbrushes in closed cupboards and rinse them before use.

Urine infections (UTI)

A UTI is very common in a toddler or young child, particularly one who is toilet training. In many cases there is no apparent cause, but it is worth knowing that two factors that can increase the risk of a UTI developing include:

- Children 'holding on' to their wee too long, even though they need to go to the toilet. This can occur as a result of nerve damage but is most commonly due to habit, which can be difficult to break. Some very shy toddlers may be too nervous or embarrassed to ask, or want to use the toilet away from home. They may hold on to their wee when they are at nursery or in a new childcare setting. Most usually grow out of this habit, as they grow more confident in a new setting and start to adopt more regular bathroom habits.

- Constipation: this can put pressure on the bladder making it more prone to infection; the bladder doesn't empty normally and the remaining urine becomes infected by bacteria. For advice on dealing with constipation, see page 215.

Causes

Most UTIs are caused by bacteria that live in the digestive system. When the bacteria gets into the urethra (the tube that urine passes through), it can cause infection. In young children this can occur when they wipe their bottom after going to the toilet and soiled paper comes into contact with their genitals.

Girls are more at risk than boys because there is less distance between their bottom and urethra. Practise teaching any girl toddlers you have to wipe from front to back, which will reduce the risk.

Symptoms

Symptoms vary depending on the age of the child. Infants older than three months but not old enough to talk:

- High temperature of 38°C (100.4°F) or above
- Abdominal pain
- Feeling of tenderness around the pelvis
- Vomiting

- Poor feeding
- Lethargy
- Irritability
- Blood in the urine
- Unpleasant-smelling urine
- Failure to thrive

In children old enough to talk:

- A frequent need to urinate
- Complaining of pain or a burning sensation during urination
- Deliberately holding in their urine
- A change in normal toilet habits, such as wetting themselves or wetting the bed
- Complaining of a feeling of tenderness around the pelvis
- Fever
- Complaining of feeling generally unwell
- Blood in the urine
- Unpleasant-smelling urine
- Cloudy urine

Treatment

Take your toddler to the GP if she develops any of the above symptoms. Most UTIs in children don't cause concern but do need to be treated with antibiotics. A urine test will be done and your GP will advise on the best course of action. If your toddler has been unwell with no obvious source of infection, e.g. sore ears or throat or a cold, it's worth taking a urine sample to the GP to ask them to check for infection.

Whooping cough

Whooping cough is a highly contagious bacterial infection of the lungs and airways. The medical term for it is Pertussis. With the UK immunisation programme in place and your child up to date on her vaccinations, it is unlikely you will have to deal with this infection. Pregnant women are now routinely offered the whooping cough vaccination after their 28th week of pregnancy to protect their unborn baby and give them some immunity, until they are old enough to have their own vaccination.

As whooping cough is highly infectious then you should keep your child away from others until she has either completed a five-day course of antibiotics or had the second stage of the infection (intense bouts of coughing) for three weeks or more. Although coughing may go on for longer than three weeks, your child is unlikely to still be infectious because the bacteria will have gone.

I have worked with two sets of twins who had whooping cough. At the time it was awful for them, and all of us involved in their care, to see them struggle and cough so much, particularly at night-time. The best remedy was always to pick them up, sit them upright and just pat and rub their backs as if we were winding them, until the coughing bout passed. Reassuring a child to keep them calm is essential and offering them a few sips of water afterwards may help. I'm happy to say that both sets of twins recovered fully with no complications!

Symptoms

Whooping cough has an incubation period of between 6–20 days, so it can take some time for symptoms to appear after initial infection with the whooping cough bacteria. It tends to develop in stages, with mild symptoms first, followed by more severe symptoms and then improvement.

Early symptoms are similar to those of a common cold and can last for 1–2 weeks before becoming worse:

- Dry, irritating cough
- Runny or blocked nose
- Slightly raised temperature
- Sore throat
- Sneezing
- Watering eyes
- Feeling generally unwell

The second stage of whooping cough causes intense bouts of coughing, sometimes referred to as 'paroxysms' of coughing. This may include:

- Intense coughing bouts, which bring up thick phlegm
- A 'whoop' sound with each sharp intake of breath after coughing (although this may not occur in infants and young children). Infants younger than six months may instead start gagging or gasping and may even temporarily stop breathing. Young children may also seem to choke or become blue in the face when they have a bout of coughing. This often looks worse than it is and breathing will quickly restart again, although of course if you are worried then seek urgent medical attention.
- Vomiting after coughing, especially in infants and young children
- Tiredness and redness in the face from the effort of coughing

- Each bout of coughing usually lasts 1–2 minutes but several bouts may occur in quick succession and last several minutes. The number of coughing bouts each day can vary but it is usually between 12–15.

Treatment

If whooping cough is diagnosed during the first 21 days of the infection, your GP may prescribe antibiotics to help prevent the infection spreading to others. If your child is not diagnosed until the later stages of the infection, it's unlikely your GP will prescribe antibiotics as they will not actually improve symptoms. Babies under one year are often admitted to hospital for monitoring. Whooping cough is much less serious in children over one year old, older children and adults. Your GP will usually advise self-help measures to manage the infection at home:

- Offer lots of fluids to prevent dehydration
- Rest
- Give infant ibuprofen and/or infant paracetamol to relieve a high temperature or sore throat
- Wipe excess mucus or vomit during bouts of coughing with a tissue, towel or warm flannel so it cannot be inhaled and cause choking

All of the information provided in this chapter regarding symptoms and treatment was correct at the time of writing. Although the advice is here to help you, if you have any concerns about your child at any time when unwell or displaying certain symptoms, always seek medical attention for a confirmed diagnosis.

9
Developmental milestones

As a baby develops into a toddler, developmental milestones are assessed over a longer timeframe. Instead of being within a 1–3-month range, a toddler's key areas are observed over a much longer period of time. As long as toddlers can meet certain targets within that timescale, their development is deemed normal.

When your toddler begins pre-school or nursery, the Early Years Foundation Stage (EYFS) requires all early years practitioners to review each child's progress and share a summary with the parents. This should happen between the ages of 24–36 months via the progress check and again at the end of the primary school reception year, via the EYFS profile.

The Early Years Outcomes is a non-statutory guide to support practitioners. It can be used by childminders, nurseries, pre-schools and any childcare setting that is inspected by Ofsted (see page 201) throughout the early years, as a guide to judging whether children are showing typical development for their age, may be at risk of delay or are ahead for their age.

Pre-school or nursery staff are advised to provide additional support to help children meet those targets when necessary and a need has been identified. Rather than give you a set of developmental milestones based on another set of guidelines, I thought it would be helpful for you to have details of the key areas of development that your toddler's other carers will be concentrating on and observing, when he begins to attend a regular childcare setting. This will help you all encourage and stimulate him with consistency, to aid his progress in the best way possible. If there is a problem with a particular area of development. it will be easier to identify and discuss with your child's key worker at nursery and plan how to move forward.

The sections below set out what you should be able to observe a child doing at each stage if he is developing normally for his age. The age ranges are spread across 14–20 months as a typical period within which a child can hit a particular milestone. This vast timeframe of what is still deemed 'normal development' should hopefully reassure you. Siblings and twins within the same family can still hit their milestones within a normal range, even if they achieve them a few months apart.

You will notice that the age ranges overlap too. This is because children develop different skills at certain times within a set period, but are still within a normal range of development. Even if toddlers don't vocalise as early or develop certain physical skills as their peers did, for the most part they all catch up eventually. In general, by the age of five years old, when children reach reception in primary school, their key areas of development are usually on par with their peers.

To keep in line with my first book, I have split the milestones into three sections and included what you can do to encourage your toddler to develop the skills necessary to hit their milestones.

- **Beginner skills:** The behaviour and things toddlers can do at the younger end of the age range stated.

- **Intermediate skills:** The skills and behaviour toddlers begin to achieve as they improve and are encouraged in a particular skill or activity.
- **Advanced skills:** Skills and behaviour toddlers are able to do easily all the time.

22–36 months
Beginner skills

- Listens with interest to the noises adults make when they read stories
- Recognises and responds to many familiar sounds – for example, turns when he hears a knock on the door, looks at or goes to the door
- Shows an interest in play when he hears sounds, songs and rhymes being used and wants to join in
- Identifies action words by pointing to the right picture – for example, 'Who's jumping?'
- Uses his developing language as a way of engaging and playing with new children, and explaining how he feels and his thoughts and experiences
- Runs safely on the whole of his foot, rather than running on tip toes as a younger toddler might
- Squats with steadiness to rest or play with an object on the ground and rises to his feet without using his hands
- Climbs confidently and begins to pull himself up on climbing equipment
- Can kick a large ball
- Turns pages in a book, sometimes several at once
- Shows control in holding and using jugs to pour
- Enjoys banging or hammering with various objects and tools
- Uses books and mark-making tools, such as pencils, pens and chalk

- Feeds himself completely with a spoon
- Drinks from a cup with no lid well without spilling
- Expresses his preferences and interests
- Seeks comfort from familiar adults when needed
- Can express his own feelings such as sad, happy, cross, scared or worried
- Is aware that some actions can hurt or harm others
- Shows affection and concern for people who are special to him
- Has some favourite stories, rhymes, songs, poems or jingles
- Recites some numbers in sequence
- Uses some language to describe quantities such as 'more' and 'a lot'
- Understands some talk about immediate past and future, e.g. 'before', 'later' or 'soon'
- Anticipates specific time-based events, such as mealtimes or home time
- Has a sense of his own immediate family relations
- In pretend play, he imitates everyday activities and events from his own family and cultural background – for example, making and drinking tea
- Enjoys playing with small world models such as a farm, garage or train track
- Wants to learn the basic skills to turn on and operate equipment
- Creates sounds by banging, shaking, tapping or blowing
- Experiments with blocks, colours and making marks using crayons and pencils
- Begins to use representation to communicate – for example, drawing a line and saying, 'That's me!'

Intermediate skills

- Understands more complex sentences – for example, 'Put your toys away and then we'll read a book'
- Holds a conversation, jumping from topic to topic
- Learns new words very rapidly and is able to use them in communicating
- Uses gestures, sometimes with limited talk – for example, reaches towards a toy saying 'I have it'
- Begins to use three fingers (tripod grip) to hold writing tools
- Imitates drawing simple shapes, such as circles and lines
- Walks upstairs or downstairs holding on to a rail, two feet to a step
- Clearly communicates his need for the potty or toilet
- Begins to recognise danger and seeks support of significant adults for help
- Separates from main carer, with support and encouragement from a familiar adult
- Helps with clothing – for example, puts on a hat, unzips a jacket, takes off unbuttoned shirt
- Aware that some actions can hurt or harm others
- Tries to help or give comfort when others are distressed
- Shows understanding and co-operates with some boundaries and routines
- Responds to the feelings and wishes of others
- Interested in others playing and starts to join in
- May form a special friendship with another child
- Repeats words or phrases from familiar stories
- Selects a small number of objects from a group when asked – for example, 'Please give me one', 'Please give me two'
- Notices simple shapes and patterns in pictures

- Begins to categorise objects according to properties, such as shape or size
- Begins to use the language of size
- Begins to have his own friends
- Operates mechanical toys – for example, turns the knob on a wind-up toy or pulls back a friction car
- Joins in singing favourite songs
- Begins to make-believe by pretending

Advanced skills

- Can shift to a different task if his attention is fully obtained – using the child's name helps him to focus
- Understands 'who', 'what', 'where' in simple questions – for example, 'Who's that?', 'What's that?', 'Where is?'
- Develops an understanding of simple concepts – for example, big/little
- Uses a variety of questions (for example, 'What?', 'Where?', 'Who?')
- Uses simple sentences – for example, 'Mummy gone work'
- May be beginning to show preference for using a dominant hand
- Beginning to be independent in self-care, like washing hands, etc., but still often needs adult support
- Distinguishes between the different marks they make on paper and will tell you what they have drawn or 'written'
- Can inhibit own actions/behaviours – for example, he stops himself from doing something he shouldn't do
- Begins to have a growing ability to distract himself when upset – for example, by engaging in a new play activity
- Seeks out others to share experiences

- Fills in the missing word or phrase in a known rhyme, story or game – for example, 'Humpty Dumpty sat on a ...'
- Creates and experiments with symbols and marks representing ideas of number, e.g. drawing eyes on a face or arms and legs on a body
- Knows that a group of things changes in quantity when something is added or taken away
- Learns that he has similarities and differences that connect them to and distinguish them from others
- Notices detailed features of objects in his own environment, e.g. on a nature trail
- Shows an interest in the way musical instruments sound

Toys, activities and parental encouragement

During this period of your toddler's development, he will have a huge amount going on and it's very important you show lots of patience, as that will make all the transitions he has to make so much easier for him, you and the rest of the family. Starting a nursery or pre-school, beginning toilet training and learning about the different boundaries each parent, as well as other childcarers, expect to be followed, can mean he may become frustrated on a regular basis.

He will be learning new skills in all areas of his development and you can aid that and encourage him along the way by being very patient. Provide opportunities for him to practise the physical skills he is interested in most at this age – drawing, play dough, climbing, running and jumping, as well as doing puzzles. Meet up with friends who have babies of a similar age and younger babies and go to toddler groups, so that your child can be taught and encouraged to play co-operatively with others and be kind and gentle during play.

Talk to him about anything and everything you and he do together, as well as past events and things you may be planning to do. During this period of development his language skills will increase on a weekly basis with new words being learnt daily, so encourage this as much as you can. Don't worry too much about his pronunciation of words at this stage, as that will come more easily later on as his speech and understanding develops. Sing songs, read books together and help him widen his vocabulary even while doing everyday household tasks. Everything is an opportunity to learn at this age and your toddler will be eager to be involved.

30 to 50 months
Beginner skills

- Listens to others one to one or in small groups, when conversation interests him
- Listens to stories with increasing attention and recall
- Responds to simple instructions – for example, to get or put away an object
- Builds up vocabulary that reflects the breadth of his experiences
- Uses vocabulary focused on objects and people that are of particular importance to him
- Can retell a simple past event in correct order – for example, went down slide, hurt finger
- Uses language to pretend that an object stands for something else in play – for example, 'This box is my castle'
- Can stand momentarily on one foot when shown
- Can catch a large ball
- Walks downstairs two feet to each step while carrying a small object

- Can usually manage washing and drying hands
- Dresses with help – for example, puts arms into open-fronted coat or shirt when held up, pulls up own trousers and pulls zipper once it is fastened at the bottom
- Can tell adults when he is hungry or tired or when he wants to rest or play
- Can select and use activities and resources with help
- Welcomes and values praise for what he has done
- Enjoys the responsibility of carrying out small tasks
- Aware of own feelings and knows that some actions and words can hurt others' feelings
- Keeps play going by responding to what others are saying or doing
- Enjoys rhyming and rhythmic activities
- Listens to stories with increasing attention and recall
- Looks at books independently
- Listens to and joins in with stories and poems one-to-one and also in small groups
- Sometimes gives meaning to marks as he draws and paints
- Recites numbers in order to 10
- Knows that numbers identify how many objects are in a set
- Shows curiosity about numbers by offering comments or asking questions
- Shows an interest in shape and space by playing with shapes or making arrangements with objects
- Shows an interest in shapes in the environment, such as shapes of windows, doors and car wheels
- Shows interest in the lives of people who are familiar to him
- Remembers and talks about significant events in his own experiences

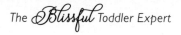

- Can talk about some of the things he has observed, such as plants, animals, natural and found objects
- Shows care and concern for living things and the environment
- Knows how to operate simple equipment, such as a child's interactive toy or a laptop/tablet; can turn on the TV and press a light switch
- Shows an interest in technological toys with knobs or pulleys or real objects
- Enjoys joining in with dancing and ring games, such as 'Ring a Ring o' Roses' and 'Hokey Cokey'
- Sings a few familiar songs
- Begins to move rhythmically
- Imitates movement in response to music
- Develops preferences for forms of expression
- Uses movement to express feelings
- Creates movement in response to music
- Sings to self and makes up simple songs

Intermediate skills

- Joins in with repeated words and anticipates key events and phrases in rhymes and stories – for example *We're Going on a Bear Hunt'* or *Dear Zoo*
- Focusing attention but can still listen or do – for example, can have a conversation with another child while doing a puzzle
- Understands use of objects – for example, knows a knife is used to cut things
- Shows understanding of prepositions such as 'under', 'on top', 'behind' by carrying out an action or selecting the correct picture

- Uses intonation, rhythm and phrasing to make the meaning clear to others
- Draws circles and lines using gross motor movements
- Uses one-handed tools and equipment – for example, makes snips in paper with child scissors
- Holds pencil between thumb and two fingers, no longer using whole-hand grasp
- Mounts stairs, steps or climbing equipment using alternate feet
- Observes the effects of activity on his body – for example, he recognises that running or jumping has an effect on his energy levels, how hot he feels and how fast his heart beats
- Understands that equipment and tools have to be used safely
- Confident to talk to other children when playing and will communicate freely about his own home and community
- Begins to accept the needs of others and can take turns and share resources, sometimes with support from others
- Can play in a group, extending and elaborating play ideas – for example, building up a role-play activity with other children
- Handles books carefully
- Knows information can be relayed in the form of print
- Holds books the correct way up and turns pages
- Suggests how the story might end
- Shows awareness of rhyme and alliteration
- When he speaks, he now recognises that some words rhyme
- Beginning to be aware of the way stories are structured
- Shows an interest in number problems – for example, which group of objects has the most or putting numbers in order
- Separates a group of three or four objects in different ways, beginning to recognise that the total is still the same

- Compares two groups of objects, saying when there is the same number of items in each
- Shows an interest in representing numbers – for example, he draws a certain number of objects when asked to
- Shows an interest in numbers in the environment around him – for example, he points out the numbers on a bus, the house numbers on doors, etc
- Realises not only objects, but anything can be counted, including steps, claps or jumps
- Uses shapes appropriately for tasks
- Begins to talk about the shapes or sizes of everyday objects – for example 'round' and 'tall'
- Shows awareness of similarities of shapes in the environment – for example, he notices that a car's wheel is a circle or a window is a square
- Recognises and describes special times or events for family or friends
- Shows interest in different occupations and ways of life
- Comments and asks questions about aspects of his familiar world, such as the place where he lives or the natural world
- Knows that information can be retrieved from computers
- Taps out simple repeated rhymes
- Explores and learns how sounds can be changed
- Explores colour and how colours can be changed
- Understands that he can use lines to enclose a space and then begin to use those shapes to represent objects – for example, he draws a square to represent a house
- Begins to be interested in and describe the texture of things
- Uses various construction materials
- Makes up rhythms by banging or tapping with musical instruments or basic household objects, such as saucepans or cups

- Notices what adults do, imitating what is observed and then doing it spontaneously when the adult is not there
- Engages in imaginative role-play based on own first-hand experiences

Advanced skills

- Is able to follow directions (if not intently focused on his own choice of activity)
- Begins to understand 'why' and 'how' questions
- Questions why things happen and gives explanations. Asks 'Who?', 'What?', 'When?', 'How?'
- Uses a range of tenses – for example, play, playing, will play, played
- Begins to use more complex sentences to link thoughts – for example, using 'and' and 'because'
- Uses speech to connect ideas, explain what is happening and anticipate what might happen next, and to recall and relive past experiences
- Holds a pencil near the point, between his first two fingers and thumb, and uses it with good control
- Can copy some letters – for example, letters from his name
- Moves freely and with pleasure and confidence in a range of ways, such as slithering, shuffling, rolling, crawling, walking, running, jumping, skipping, sliding and hopping
- Runs skilfully and negotiates space successfully, adjusting his speed and direction to avoid obstacles
- Gains more bowel and bladder control and can attend to toileting needs most of the time himself
- Is more outgoing towards unfamiliar people and more confident in new social situations
- Shows confidence in asking adults for help

- Can usually tolerate delay when his needs are not immediately met and understands that his wishes may not always be met
- Can usually adapt his behaviour to different events, social situations and changes in routine
- Initiates play, offering cues for his peers to join in
- Demonstrates friendly behaviour, initiating conversations and forming good relationships with peers and familiar adults
- Describes main story settings, events and principal characters
- Shows an interest in illustrations and print in books and print in the environment
- Recognises familiar words and signs, such as his own name and advertising logos
- Knows that print carries meaning and, in English, is read from left to right and top to bottom
- Ascribes meaning to marks that he sees in different places – seeing his name or a familiar supermarket brand, for example
- Uses some number names and number language spontaneously – for example, 'I have three bricks. Please can I have more?'
- Uses some number names accurately in play
- Begins to represent numbers using fingers, marks on paper or pictures
- Sometimes matches numeral and quantity correctly
- Uses positional language, such as 'first' and 'last'
- Shows an interest in shape by wanting to construct or build things using Lego or bricks, for example
- Knows some of the things that make him unique and can talk about some of the similarities and differences in relation to friends and family, such as eye and hair colour

- Talks about why things happen and how things work
- Develops an understanding of growth, decay and changes over time – for example, food that goes bad if not eaten, the leaves changing in the autumn
- Shows skill in making toys work by pressing parts or lifting flaps to achieve effects such as sound, movements or new images
- Begins to construct, stacking blocks vertically and horizontally, making enclosures and creating spaces
- Joins construction pieces together to build and balance
- Realises tools can be used for a purpose
- Builds stories around toys – for example, his toy farm animals need to be rescued from an armchair 'cliff'
- Uses available resources to create props to support role-play
- Captures experiences and responses with a range of media, such as music, dance and paint and other materials or words

Toys, activities and parental encouragement

During this period of development, your toddler will have a very active imagination and enjoy using it to role-play and make the toys and activities he is involved in more interesting. Encourage that by setting up small world activities, such as a doll's house, or a car or train track, or even by just letting him try various dressing-up clothes on and pretending he is off somewhere special, or has a particular job. Join in to help broaden his imagination and give him new ideas, which he will remember next time.

He will begin to be more interested in drawing pictures and writing words that mean something now, rather than the early scribbles he used to be happy doing. You can begin to talk about numbers and letters and the sounds they make, and

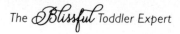

how to write them down on paper. At this age toddlers enjoy trying to follow the dots, so you can mark out the dots of his name on a piece of paper and encourage him to follow them with his pencil or crayon.

He will also begin to have much more interest in the world around him, outside of his immediate family – he may be interested in other people and ask about things he sees and how they work. Try to answer simply but as honestly as you can, even if the questions you are asked are sometimes embarrassing. Children begin to notice that there are lots of different people in the world and some look very different. Help him to understand that this is okay and he will grow up accepting people's differences as normal.

40– 60 months+

Beginner skills

- Maintains attention, concentrates and sits quietly during appropriate activity
- Introduces a storyline or narrative into play
- Experiments with different ways of moving
- Jumps off an object and can land safely
- Uses simple tools to effect changes to materials – for example, cutting paper with scissors
- Usually dry and clean during the day but not necessarily at night
- Aware of the boundaries set and of behavioural expectations in a childcare setting
- Uses vocabulary and forms of speech that are increasingly influenced by his experience of books
- Enjoys an increasing range of books
- Knows that information can be retrieved from books and computers

- Gives meaning to marks he makes as he draws, writes and paints
- Continues a rhyming string – for example 'cat, sat, mat'
- Hears and says the initial sound in words – for example, 'h for Harry', 'm for Mummy'
- Recognises some numerals of personal significance – for example, his own age or house number
- Recognises numerals 1–5
- Counts up to three or four objects by saying one number name for each item, while pointing to them individually and stopping once all have been counted
- Counts actions or objects that cannot be moved, such as stairs
- Uses everyday language related to time – for example, lunchtime, today, slow, fast, now, soon
- Beginning to use everyday language related to money
- Orders and sequences familiar events – things that happen during the day and their order: breakfast, going to the shops, home, lunch, play, bathtime, bedtime
- Measures short periods of time in simple ways
- Enjoys joining in with family customs and routines
- Begins to build a repertoire of songs and dances
- Explores the different sounds of instruments
- Explores what happens when he mixes colours
- Chooses a particular colour to use for a purpose
- Plays alongside other children who are engaged in the same theme

Intermediate skills
- Has two-channelled attention – can listen and do for a short amount of time

- Responds to instructions that involve a two-part sequence
- Able to follow a story without pictures or props
- Uses language to imagine and recreate roles and experiences in play situations
- Links statements, and sticks to a main theme or intention
- Shows understanding of how to transport and store equipment safely
- Practises some appropriate safety measures without direct supervision, such as walking down the stairs carefully
- Understands that his actions affect other people – for example, becomes upset or tries to comfort another child when he realises he has upset them
- Initiates conversations, attends to and takes account of what others say
- Hears and says the initial sound in words – for example, 'm for Mummy', 'd for Daddy'
- Begins to break the flow of speech into words and blend them together, spelling out words using the letter sounds – for example, C-A-T
- Links sounds to letters, naming and sounding the letters of the alphabet
- Counts objects to 10 and begins to count beyond 10
- Counts out up to six objects from a larger group
- Selects the correct numeral to represent 1–5, then 1–10 objects
- Counts an irregular arrangement of up to 10 objects
- Measures short periods of time in simple ways – for example, 'It's my birthday tomorrow.' 'We will be having lunch after we have been to the shop.'
- Uses familiar objects and common shapes to create and recreate patterns and build models

- Interacts with age-appropriate computer software
- Experiments to create different textures – for example, by cooking or doing a play dough activity
- Understands that different materials can be combined to create new effects – for example, being involved in a messy play activity like painting or sand and water mixed together
- Constructs with a purpose in mind, using a variety of resources – for example, junk modelling, play dough, Lego
- Plays co-operatively as part of a group to develop and act out a narrative

Advanced skills

- Listens and responds to ideas expressed by others in conversation or discussion
- Understands humour – for example, nonsense rhymes and simple jokes
- Extends vocabulary, especially by grouping and naming, exploring the meaning and sounds of new words
- Uses speech to organise, sequence and clarify thinking, ideas, feelings and events
- Negotiates space successfully when playing racing and chasing games with other children, adjusting his speed or changing direction to avoid obstacles
- Travels with confidence and skill around, under, over and through balancing and climbing equipment
- Shows increasing control over an object in pushing, patting, throwing, catching or kicking it
- Handles tools, objects, construction and malleable materials safely and with increasing control
- Shows a preference for a dominant hand

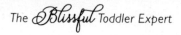

- Begins to use anti-clockwise movement and retrace vertical lines
- Begins to use a pencil effectively to write recognisable letters, most of which are correctly formed
- Shows some understanding that good practices with regard to exercise, eating, sleeping and hygiene contribute to good health
- Shows understanding of the need for safety when tackling new challenges, and considers and manages some risks
- Is confident to speak to others about own needs, wants, interests and opinions
- Can describe himself in positive terms and talk about his abilities
- Begins to be able to negotiate and solve problems without aggression – for example, when another child has taken his toy
- Explains his own knowledge and understands and asks appropriate questions of others
- Takes steps to resolve conflicts with other children by finding a compromise
- Can segment the sounds in simple words and blend them together and knows which letters represent some of them – for example, spelling the word D-O-G using the letter sounds
- Links sounds to letters, naming and sounding the letters of the alphabet
- Begins to read words and simple sentences
- Can now write some clearly identifiable letters to communicate meaning, representing some sounds correctly and in sequence

- Writes own name and other things such as basic words under pictures he may draw, e.g. CAT under a picture of a cat he's drawn
- Estimates how many objects he can see and checks by counting them
- Uses the language of 'more' and 'less' to compare two sets of objects
- Finds the total number of items in two groups by counting all of them
- Says the number that is one more than a given number, so if you ask 'What is after 5?' then he should answer '6'!
- In practical activities and discussion, begins to use the vocabulary involved in adding and subtracting
- Begins to identify own mathematical problems based on own interests and fascinations – for example, he knows that he doesn't have enough bricks to build a Lego house
- Attempts to write short sentences in meaningful contexts – for example, 'The cat sat on the mat'
- Begins to use mathematical names for 'solid' 3D shapes and 'flat' 2D shapes and mathematical terms such as 'pyramid' and 'cube' to describe shapes
- Selects a particular named shape
- Can describe a relative position, such as 'behind' or 'next to'
- Can put two or three items in order by length or height
- Can put two items in order by weight or capacity
- Looks closely at similarities, differences, patterns and change
- Completes a simple programme on a computer, such as a child's interactive game on a tablet app or website
- Uses simple tools and techniques, such as cutting, sticking with a glue stick, painting or even writing competently and appropriately

- Selects appropriate resources to use when completing an activity but can adapt and choose alternative things to use if the activity is not going well – for example, getting a new pen if the current one doesn't work or runs out
- Selects tools and technique needed to shape, assemble and join materials he is using – for example, when making a collage at home, he will know that he needs paper, glue, scissors and pictures to stick on
- Creates simple representations of events, people and objects
- Initiates new combinations of movement and gesture in order to express and respond to feelings, ideas and experiences – for example, showing compassion if a friend or someone close to him is upset and offering comfort

Toys, activities and parental encouragement

This is the age you need to begin preparing your child for starting school. Encourage him to sit down with you and be involved in structured learning activities, so he doesn't find that too difficult when he starts school. It's important to make things fun, though, so he enjoys what you are doing and is able to learn new skills and practise current ones.

If his speech and pronunciation is still a little hard to understand at times, then practise the words he is struggling with to get the beginning sounds correct. Help him become independent and ensure he can go to the toilet for both a wee and poo by himself and dress and undress without help, in preparation for changing into a P.E. kit at school. There will, of course, always be people to help at school, but your child will feel much more relaxed and confident in an already new situation with lots of new people, if he can manage to do most things without help.

All of the above information is available for download at www.gov.uk/government/publications and is accurate and dated September 2013 as the most recent publication at the time this book went to print.

I hope that having an idea of the guidelines your toddler's childcare setting will be using will be helpful. As a mother of a toddler myself, I have actually enjoyed reading the different types of behaviour and matching up which ones my little girl can already do and which areas we can work on. Please be aware, as already previously stated, that many things can impact the speed at which a child develops and hits their milestones:

- Position in the family
- A major change that happens during the toddler years – for example, a new sibling, house move, family dynamics changing due to divorce or death
- Work commitments and making quality time

Helping your child's development

A chance to practise and develop new skills will make the major difference to how quickly and easily your toddler hits the early learning goals. Helping to build his confidence as he attempts new things will also play a major part. His environment and the activities and stimulation he is given at home will influence which skills he is likely to learn the fastest.

None of us are fantastic at anything the first few times we try a new activity or skill, but with repetition, patience and perseverance, we can all get better at doing things.

Your job as a parent is to provide your toddler with a safe, stimulating environment where he can try new things and

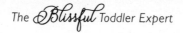

develop them and, as long as he's given the right opportunities, he will naturally improve in the key areas and meet all the learning goals expected for his age.

If he is struggling, it is worth having a chat with his key worker at nursery, or other childcare setting he is attending, and ask if they have noticed the same issues or have any concerns. Together you can make a plan to encourage skills that may be lacking and they will also be able to advise if they think there may be a developmental problem that you need to discuss further with a health professional.

Remember, for the most part, once children reach primary school age, they will be 'on par' with their peers and within a normal expected range of development, so try not to worry (too much)!

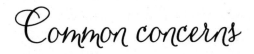

Common concerns

At what age should I begin toilet training?
There is no specific age to begin toilet training. It's about noticing signs that your toddler is ready. This usually happens between the ages of 2–3 years old, but can be earlier with some toddlers and later with others. Full details of the signs and how to toilet train without stress can be found in Chapter 6.

How many words should my two-year-old be saying?
Understanding comes before actual speech and although your toddler may still have fewer than 50 words in her total vocabulary, she will understand many more and be able to follow a range of instructions you give, such as 'Put that in the bin' and 'Fetch me the ball.' By two years she may be starting to string two words together, such as 'Up please'. All children develop speech at different stages of their toddlerhood and there are many factors that can influence it, as discussed in more detail in Chapter 4.

My 18-month-old has started to have tantrums already. How do I deal with this?
Early tantrums are usually linked to toddlers being frustrated by not having the words to express what they want easily or

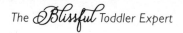

make themselves understood. Your toddler is also learning that he can't always have everything he wants. Distraction is the best way to deal with an impending tantrum or one that has started. Interest him in another activity or make something else seem like the most wonderful thing you have ever seen to take his mind off whatever was causing his frustration. He will very quickly forget about the thing that wound him up in the first place. You will find more tips and ways to deal with tantrums in Chapter 3.

How much sleep should my toddler have? At what age will she drop her daytime nap?

Toddlers still need 11–13 hours' sleep per night. It varies as to what age a toddler will no longer need a nap – some will drop it at two years old, but others still need a daytime nap at 3–4 years. Be guided by the needs of your child. As long as she still settles and sleeps well at bedtime and overnight, a nap over the lunchtime period will benefit her and help to stop her becoming overtired and fractious in the afternoon and evening. If your toddler is a poor sleeper anyway, read Chapter 1 to find out the possible reasons and how to encourage better overnight sleep.

What age should I transition my toddler from a cot to a bed?

Again, there is no specific age. Be guided by when your child is showing readiness to move out of his cot. If he is climbing out of his cot every time you put him in it, a transition to a cot sooner rather than later is essential for his safety. If he is quite happily sleeping in his cot still at two years old, my recommendation is to wait until sometime around the age of two-and-a-half before making the transition. At that age, your toddler's speech and understanding should be improving and it will be much easier to explain what is happening to him and also encourage him to want to settle and stay in his bed, rather than get out frequently now he knows that's an option. More details on making the transition from cot to bed can be found on page 17.

How do I prepare my toddler for the arrival of a new baby?
There are many things you can do to help prepare your toddler for a baby sibling to ensure the new arrival is not too disruptive and only a positive thing for your toddler to enjoy. See pages 119–25 for lots of information on this and some tips for before and after the baby is born.

When should I move my toddler from formula/breast-feeding to cow's milk?
Cow's milk can be given to drink any time from the age of 12 months. If you would prefer to continue breastfeeding or use the toddler formula milk after 12 months that is, of course, fine and your own personal choice.

How much milk should my toddler be drinking per day?
Children between the ages of one and three need to have around 350 mg of calcium a day. About 300 ml (just over half a pint) of milk would provide this. If your toddler is having dairy in other forms, such as cheese and yoghurts, you can reduce his daily intake of milk.

My toddler says 'No' all the time whenever I ask him to do something. How do I deal with this?
This is a normal part of his development and speech process. He learns that he can have a choice in things now he's getting

older and makes every attempt to make himself and his wants known. Try to give choices between two things in almost everything you do, so that he feels he has some control. This will make life a lot easier and less stressful for both of you, as he will feel like he has choices and you will be providing him options between two things you are happy for him to choose from. Distraction and lots of enthusiasm are other tools that will help you convince him to do things he's not so keen on.

How can I help my toddler develop her speech?

In short, talk to her all the time about anything and everything! Babies and toddlers learn by example and the more she hears you talk, the more her understanding will develop and in turn her speech. Read the tips in Chapter 4 for more details on how to do this and what activities will help.

How can I encourage my toddler to share and be kind?

Be a good role model. She will mimic how you behave, so if she sees you talking nicely and being kind and helpful to others she will naturally follow suit. Encourage role-play with a doll or teddy. Play with it in pretend situations to show her how to be kind and share. Take her to toddler groups and meet up with friends regularly. The more she mixes with her peers, the better she will become at understanding how to share and watching others do it will help too. For more information see Chapter 3.

My toddler can sometimes be aggressive with other children and try to bite them! How should I deal with it?

Try to work out what triggers the aggression. In toddlers it usually stems from frustration and an inability to express their feelings or what they want due to their limited language skills at this age. It can also be something they do if they are teething particularly badly as they need something to mouth to ease the pain. More details on how to prevent and react to biting can be found on page 100.

Each time I try to strap my son into his buggy or car seat he has a tantrum and it's very difficult to get him in at all! He's very strong! How do I deal with this?

Distraction is the best way to deal with this. Try giving him something to eat or drink or chat or sing to him as you strap him in, or point out a really exciting object, animal or person you see close by. These activities can be enough to distract him while you quickly strap him in before be realises what's happening!

How do I transition from two naps (morning and afternoon) down to one nap and fit meals in?

The ideal time to encourage a nap once you drop down to one per day is over the lunchtime period. This usually needs to happen around the age of 12–15 months. You will know your toddler is ready to drop to one nap as he will become difficult to settle for his usual morning and afternoon naps and/or begin to take very short naps, even though he is clearly still tired. To begin with your toddler will struggle to get past 12pm, so you need to give an early lunch around 11:20/30am and then put him straight to bed afterwards for around 2–3 hours. Always ensure he is awake by 3pm if you want him to settle well for a 7/7:30pm bedtime As he gets a little older and able to stay awake a bit longer, you can begin to push his lunch

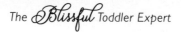

and nap a little later so he can have lunch around 12pm and a nap straight after.

What is the correct portion size to give to my toddler at mealtimes?

To begin with give a portion the size of your clenched fist. Putting too much food on to your toddler's plate initially may overwhelm her and put her off even attempting the meal. You can always offer more if she finishes the first helping and asks for extra.

Do I need to give my toddler vitamin drops?

The current advice from the Department of Health (at the time of writing) is that all babies and toddlers from six months to five years should be given supplements in the form of vitamin drops, which contain vitamins A, C and D. Children who do not eat a varied diet don't always get enough of vitamins A and C, and vitamin D is only found naturally in oily fish and eggs, with its main source being summer sunlight on your child's skin. Babies or toddlers who are still having infant formula will *not* need vitamin D supplements until they are drinking less than 500 ml (1 pint) of milk per day as their infant formula is fortified with vitamin D.

When should I start brushing my toddler's teeth?

You should ideally start brushing your child's teeth as soon as the first ones cut. If you make this part of your daily routine, you shouldn't have any issues or reluctance from your toddler. If your toddler isn't keen, it's worth allowing him to choose a special toothbrush from the wide range available now. Electric ones can have an exciting appeal or if your toddler doesn't like the noise they make, try a flashing one that gives a cue as to how long he needs to brush for. Use a reward chart to praise your toddler for having his teeth brushed if it's not an activity he's keen on doing.

Since my toddler started walking he is into everything and always trying to touch everything in the house I don't want him to! How can I make the house safe for him and teach him not to touch?

There are some things you will need to put out of his reach for his safety, but generally distraction is your best tool. If he does try to touch something that's unsafe immediately distract him with another activity to stop him being tempted to keep touching and it turning into a 'Yes–No' battle. More tips and advice can be found in Chapter 3.

My toddler wakes frequently at night. We are considering moving her to a bed to see if this will improve sleep but not sure what to do?

Moving her to a bed will not usually improve sleep. If anything her sleep issue will get worse once she realises she can get out whenever she wants to. You need to figure out the reason for the frequent waking. Can she self-settle without the help of you cuddling, rocking or staying with her? Does she use a dummy? If she's reliant on any help to always aid to sleep, it will always cause frequent waking as she passes through the sleep cycle – she will continue to need that same help to go back to sleep. You will find more information on how to encourage good settling and sleep habits in Chapter 1.

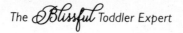

How can I encourage my twins to share and be kind to each other?

Interact with them as much as you can when they are first learning to play. Encourage sharing and kind behaviour by displaying it yourself and showing them how to share and wait their turn. Use an egg timer or something similar if there is one particular toy they both want, to give them some idea of how long they need to wait their turn. More details and tips can be found on page 102.

I am looking for a nursery for my toddler. What questions should I be asking to help me choose the right one?

There are different things that are important to different parents so the questions you ask will be relevant to your needs as a family and your individual child. For reference though there is more info in Chapter 7. Make sure you visit a few different nurseries. To begin with visit on your own without your child as it's not a good idea to unsettle your toddler with visiting lots of potential places. Once you have a shortlist of two or three, you may have an instinct for the one you like in particular. At this point arrange a visit for your toddler. Watching her reaction and how the staff interact with her is likely to be the deciding factor for you. If your toddler is happy and relaxed, that's more than half the challenge complete. Trust your instinct.

My toddler is suddenly becoming very independent and wants to do everything alone. He clearly can't always manage this, though, and gets very frustrated. What can I do to help?

Allow him to try at least and let him know that you are there to help him. Offer help initially: 'Do you want Mummy to help you?' If he says no, leave him to try. Wait to see if he's still struggling, then offer your help again. Try to give minimal help at this very independent stage but just enough to do the part that he's struggling with. If you try to allow him to finish the job off each time, he will be pleased with himself and you can praise accordingly: 'Well done, good job!'

Afterword

I hope that you have enjoyed reading my book and have found the information it has provided helpful. Remember all children have very individual personalities so the idea is for you to use the information provided and adapt it to suit you, your child and your needs at the time. If you would like more advice, you can contact me through my websites www.theblissfulbabyexpert.co.uk or www.theblissfultoddlerexpert.co.uk or post on our 'blissfulbabyclub' forum and you will receive free personalised advice.

Thank you for buying my book and good luck!

Useful resources

Visit my website www.theblissfulbabyexpert.co.uk for baby advice, product reviews and parenting forum

www.afasic.org.uk
AFASIC: Speech and Language Support Association

www.annabelkarmel.com
for information on weaning and eating

www.childcare.co.uk
for information on all aspects of childcare and how to find childcare in your local area

www.gov.uk/find-registered-childminder
to find a registered childminder

www.childrenarewelcome.co.uk
for the best child-friendly days out and places to eat for the whole family

www.elc.co.uk
Early Learning Centre for toys and play ideas

www.edspire.co.uk
for messy play ideas, reviews on toddler toys, and a blog that is truly inspirational, interesting and heart-wrenching to read

www.gltc.co.uk
Great Little Trading Company (GLTC) for toys, storage, furniture, accessories and more

www.gro.co.uk
The Gro Company for safe sleep information and products

www.gov.uk/government/publications/early-years-outcomes
Learning outcomes link to understand your child's developmental milestones

www.littlerascalsreviews.com
Review blog for parent, baby and toddler products

Mumfirstdoctorsecond.blogspot.co.uk
Blog by a mum/doctor

www.nannytax.co.uk
Nanny Tax: nanny payroll specialists

www.nannyjob.co.uk
Nannyjob: to find childcarers

www.ndna.org.uk
National Day Nurseries Association for nursery support, information and advice

www.nhs.uk/conditions/pages/hub.aspx
NHS direct website for up-to-date medical information

www.ofsted.gov.uk
The Ofsted website

Zurer Pearson, Barbara, *Raising a Bilingual Child* (Living Language, U.S., 2008)
A useful book for parents raising bilingual children

Index

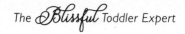

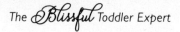

Acknowledgements

I would firstly like to thank all of the wonderful parents who I have worked alongside, with their toddlers, over the last 15 years and a special thanks to the parents who agreed to let me feature their children as case studies in this book. I'm very happy that the advice I have given has helped your family and made life much more relaxed and enjoyable for all of you.

Thank you to Emma for the lovely foreword and I look forward to helping you with your little one who is still so brand new.

I would like to thank Jessica and Caroline, who are both parents and GPs, for proofreading Chapter 8 to ensure the information I provided was accurate.

To so many friends I have met through my Twitter account and Facebook page since the launch of *The Blissful Baby Expert* and given me so much support and encouragement. I truly see you as my friends now and our online community means a lot to me. To those of you who agreed to proofread sections of the book as it was in its draft stages, I thank you for your feedback and reminders of what you wanted me to include (hopefully I remembered everything!).

To my editor Susanna, her assistant Catherine and my publicist and marketing ladies Amelia and Caitriona, thank

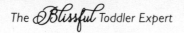

you for all your hard work behind the scenes and again making my dream of having a book published possible! I am officially an author with two books to be very proud of!

I would also like to thank my parents Jan and Des, who are a huge help and support to Martin and me. Whenever we need anything or help with the children, they are always there without question and I am grateful for their constant presence in our lives.

I must also thank my close friends and family who have encouraged me and helped me out in some way, when it all felt like a huge task ahead. I got there in the end and your support is very much appreciated.

As always, my final and greatest thanks go to my three children Jack, Ollie and Loren and my fab husband Martin. The memories we have as a family have helped me write this book and I really appreciate the support and strength you all give me with cuddles, love and fun days out, which spur me on to want to help other families work towards the same happiness. I love you all so much and I am looking forward to the next few years as many new chapters in our lives begin.

Lisa/Mummy
Xx